T0146003

"DiGregorio's storytelling is pitch-perfect; narrative and nursing, she understands, come from the same place and both are concerned with a deep understanding of character and plot.... This is a brilliant book, and DiGregorio is a beautiful writer. *Taking Care* deserves to be on the reading list for nursing and medical schools, and on the bedside table of all politicians. ... It is near impossible to articulate nursing in its vastness, yet Sarah DiGregorio has condensed its profound meaning into a call to arms."
—*New York Times Book Review*

"This probing history of nurses situates the profession as radical, necessary health care—but plagued, too, by structural inequities from sexism to racism."
—*Vanity Fair*

"In precise and approachable prose, Sarah DiGregorio uses a journalist's tools to investigate the most ethical of professions: nursing. Each chapter of *Taking Care* shows us that ethic up close—for example, when nurses advocate for women to have full access to reproductive health and for people who struggle with substance use disorder to lead purposeful lives. *Taking Care* explores how nursing has the power to make the world a better place."
—Mark Lazenby, dean and professor of the Sue & Bill Gross School of Nursing, University of California, Irvine

"*Taking Care* is a revelation. DiGregorio tracks the necessity of caretaking from neolithic times to our present moment of political struggle and climate change. Through informed hands-on care, patient advocacy, and an ongoing quest for justice, *Taking Care* shows that nurses make the world a better place."
—Theresa Brown, RN, and *New York Times* bestselling author of *Healing: When a Nurse Becomes a Patient* and *The Shift: One Nurse, Twelve Hours, Four Patients' Lives*

"In *Taking Care*, Sarah DiGregorio does the nearly impossible, seamlessly weaving together personal narratives and experiences while crafting a well-documented and researched book on the profession of nursing. DiGregorio doesn't stop with history but includes contemporary exemplars to contextualize the complexities of racism, patriarchy, and gender oppression that shaped and continue to influence the discipline. Drawing from sources across the education, clinical practice, policy, and research spectra, DiGregorio includes quotes from individuals who are nurses, work with nurses, and study nurses or nursing to create a complicated and nuanced story of the 'most trusted of the health professions.'"

—Monica R. McLemore RN, MPH, PhD,
University of Washington School of Nursing

"A capacious look at nurses throughout history, from prehistoric times to the present.... DiGregorio's abundant evidence of the crucial and transformative practice of nursing comes through her profiles of community health nurses, first responders, reproductive health providers, nurses turned politicians, and hospice nurses.... A well-informed consideration of the intimacy of care."

—*Kirkus Reviews*

"Essential reading for medical professionals or anyone interested in improving the American healthcare system, this illuminating and inspiring book shows nurses as an integral part of their communities, fighting to overcome structural inequalities such as racism, sexism, and poverty while they try to heal the nation."

—*Library Journal* (starred review)

"There are still common misconceptions about what a nurse does and what is their value to society's well-being. Sarah DiGregorio's *Taking Care* goes a long way toward countering those misconceptions and painting an accurate picture of the compassion, dedication, and knowledge that the nursing profession requires. As DiGregorio notes in her illuminating book, 'Sooner or later, we all need to be nursed.' Drawing from her own family's experiences and that of nurses both past and present, DiGregorio movingly describes nurses' historic role through the years, calling the profession 'a thread running through all human history.' This is an important book for both lay people to gain a better understanding of the work and notable contributions of nurses and to inform nurses themselves of their proud history."

—Deborah Burger, RN,
president of National Nurses United

"Powerful . . . rich and beautifully written."

—*Canadian Journal of Nursing Leadership*

"DiGregorio succeeds in offering a new, eye-opening perspective on the significance of nursing and nurses' power to better lives."

—*Booklist*

"Striking an expert balance between the big picture and intimate portraits of individual caregivers, this is an enlightening study of a crucial yet often overlooked profession."   —*Publishers Weekly*

ALSO BY SARAH DIGREGORIO

*Early: An Intimate History of Premature Birth
and What It Teaches Us About Being Human*

TAKING CARE

The Story of Nursing and Its
Power to Change Our World

Sarah DiGregorio

HARPER PERENNIAL

NEW YORK • LONDON • TORONTO • SYDNEY • NEW DELHI • AUCKLAND

HARPER ● PERENNIAL

A hardcover edition of this book was published in 2023 by Harper, an imprint of HarperCollins Publishers.

HarperCollins books may be purchased for educational, business, or sales promotional use. For information, please email the Special Markets Department at SPsales@harpercollins.com.

FIRST HARPER PERENNIAL EDITION PUBLISHED 2024.

Designed by Nancy Singer

Library of Congress Cataloging-in-Publication Data has been applied for.

ISBN 978-0-06-307129-2 (pbk.)

24 25 26 27 28 LBC 5 4 3 2 1

For Amol

And for all who nurse

CONTENTS

AUTHOR'S NOTE

I put a lot of thought into how to identify people's professional roles in this book. I would like to be succinct, clear, and respectful. In the end, I decided that the best solution was the one that would provide the most clarity for the reader with the most simplicity. So, where applicable, I have identified people upon first mention by whichever degree (PhD, MD, BSN, ADN) and license (RN, APRN, CNA) most clearly identify them within the context of this book.

Some sources have many more than two credentials, which they customarily list after their names. For those sources, I have chosen, in concert with that source, to list the degree and license best able to help the reader understand that source's role. For instance, I identify a nurse scholar who usually includes "PhD, RN, FAAN" after her name as a "PhD, RN," and then make it clear where that person works and in what context. Also, in all cases, I have omitted honorifics—including "Dr.," because it is not clarifying. (A doctor holds a doctorate. That could be a PhD, an MD, a DDS, and so on.) This is also why I refer to physicians as physicians and not doctors. By contrast, a degree and license clearly identify a person's practice, discipline, and education.

For the purposes of this book, I define nurses and nursing as broadly as possible—in part because nursing has historically been defined narrowly, in a purposefully exclusionary way with regard to race, class, gender, and cultural context. When considering practitioners over time, deciding whom to call a nurse is often subjective, as health care practices and professions have not always been defined, licensed, or delineated the way they are today. When looking to the past, I cast a wide net, including all caregivers who arguably practiced with a recognizable and distinct nursing ethos.

There are plenty of holes to be poked in this approach, but I believe that a narrower focus has only impoverished our understanding of the vast potential of nursing and served both to keep people out and to discredit different ways of knowing. This has limited the care available to everyone. Conceptualizing the field in the most expansive, inclusive ways can invite many more people into the project of nursing, help the public value nursing differently, and help nurses build new meanings from their work.

There is, of course, often a difference to be drawn between nurses who are trained and accredited and all those who "nurse." However, training and accrediting are not and have never been neutral, or available to all. When some say, for instance, that Florence Nightingale was a nurse but that her contemporary Mary Seacole, a Jamaican woman who nursed, was not, or when we call trained male nurses of the past physician assistants or orderlies instead of nurses, we are perpetuating the false idea that nurses are one kind of person, with one kind of knowing.

To find the stories in this book, I used primary sources like newspapers and autobiographies, but I also relied very much on the deep and scholarly research of nursing historians, who do the hard work of excavating and analyzing nursing history. If you are interested in nursing history, this book is a great place to start, but please note that the many historians who are quoted and cited here go deeper in their own writings than this space allows. See the extensive notes on my sources and the selected bibliography.

Quotes from the interviews I conducted have been condensed and lightly edited for clarity. In some cases—such as when a source was not authorized to speak to the press, was concerned about retaliation, or for patient privacy—interviewees are identified by their first name only, or by a pseudonym where noted.

INTRODUCTION

If you have spent any time in a hospital or health care setting, you've probably had an encounter with a nurse that lingers in your mind. For most of my life, I have accompanied my mother, my father, and my daughter, all of whom suffered serious chronic illnesses, to hospitals, clinics, and rehab centers and through therapy of all kinds. To need health care in the United States is to seek healing in what often seems to be an inhuman labyrinth. But every now and then, someone in that labyrinth manages to see you, hear you, and offer exactly what you need. For me, these encounters stand out with crystalline clarity: They were moments of relief. Someone was going to help us. Someone *could* help us—even when that help didn't include a cure; even when there wasn't a fix. And almost every single time, the person who offered what we needed was a nurse. I've come to understand that that was not a coincidence.

Sooner or later, we all need to be nursed. A nurse may have been at your birth and may be at your death; sometimes, nurses are the first and last people to touch us. Nursing is a profession, an independent scientific discipline, a practice, and a way of interacting with the world. It's also an elemental public role, one that elicits deep feelings, beliefs, and anxieties in the collective imagination.

I came to this meditation on nursing as a journalist, but also as someone who grew up surrounded by the illnesses of the people I loved most. Because I'm not a nurse myself, my perspective has limitations, but I would argue that nursing matters to everyone. It draws much of its power and effectiveness from the relationship between nurse and patient; it is the indispensable foundation of all health care. And so, in that sense, nursing *belongs* to everyone. When I was lost in the wilds of the American health care system, nurses showed me and my family how to move forward. Nurses are not just *there* at the most profound moments in people's lives; they use their knowledge and skills to *guide people through* those moments.

There was the nurse who held me by the shoulders after I ran out of my mother's hospital room, terrified. That nurse explained that the ragged, irregular gasps coming from my mother were a normal part of dying. I was twenty-one years old, alone, confused, and frightened, but that nurse told me what was happening and what to expect. She said I could stay and hold my mother's hand while the gasps got farther and farther apart and then finally stopped. She gave me and my mother the gift of being together at that moment.

There was the nurse who kept her hand on my leg when, two decades after my mother died of breast cancer, I had a suspicious mass in my own breast biopsied. While the pathologist examined the extracted cells, this nurse kept up a gentle patter, telling me about her family, how she and her two sisters had grown up in a tiny one-bedroom apartment in Manhattan, how they still liked to be physically close to one another. When the physician poked his head into the room to report that the mass was benign, the nurse put both her hands on my back and told me to feel what I needed to feel. I cried with relief.

There was the nurse with long braids who let me hug her while I got an epidural before an emergency C-section. Afterward, there was the nurse who got down next to my wheelchair and showed me how to hand-express breast milk—she literally milked me—so I could bring colostrum to my prematurely newborn daughter, Mira, who was two floors below, in the neonatal intensive care unit (NICU).

There was the NICU nurse who stood quietly and looked at Mira in her incubator for many minutes at a time. She wasn't focusing on Mira's test results or her vital signs on the monitor above. Watchful and silent, she took the time to observe minor changes in my daughter's skin tone, her arm and leg movements—just the way she *seemed* that day. It was this nurse who helped me to see my daughter underneath all the technology keeping her alive.

Then there was the visiting nurse who came to our apartment to weigh Mira every day for two weeks after she was finally discharged into a cold, anxious February. That nurse assured me that, by the time summer came, we'd be hanging out in the park with a healthy baby. She'd seen it so many times before, she said with confidence. She seemed so certain, so not shocked by my tiny baby, that she yanked me out of my own shock. And she was right—Mira improved; summer came.

The winter Mira was four years old, she struggled with asthma flare-ups. She would come into our bedroom in the dead of night gasping and wheezing, unable to speak. Before either of us was fully conscious, my husband or I would grab the rescue inhaler, press the mask to her face, and count her respiratory rate. After a few months of this, her pulmonologist decided that Mira needed a bronchoscopy, a scoped examination of her bronchial tubes and lungs to try to figure out why the standard controller treatments weren't working. My husband and I sat in the waiting room as the procedure was done under general anesthesia. It was supposed to be routine outpatient surgery—but it was taking too long. By the time they said we could come back to the recovery area, I knew something was wrong.

The attending pulmonologist rushed at me: He was on his way somewhere else; he was in a hurry. He said, "Severe, uncontrolled asthma. Lots of mucus and swelling. Bronchial tubes thirty percent smaller than expected. Airway very reactive to the procedure." And then he was gone.

Mira was still unconscious, with an oxygen mask over her face— too pale, so tiny in the hospital bed. On the monitor, her oxygen saturations were in the low- to mid-80s—too low. There were several busy clinicians in the room, including a respiratory therapist, who put Mira on a CPAP (continuous positive airway pressure) machine.

"We need to get her saturations up," someone said.

"Are you going to intubate her?" I asked the room. I heard my voice rise high with panic.

"That's one possibility," someone said.

Mira's small chest heaved, but her face was slack. Fear clamped my throat.

And then a nurse who was standing by the bed with one hand resting lightly atop Mira's head looked me right in the face. Within the hubbub of the room, she remained still, and held eye contact. With authority, she said, "It's okay, Mom. It's okay. It looks worse than it is. We're going to get her saturations up."

Throughout the next hours, that nurse never failed to look me in the eye. She never failed to talk about my daughter as my daughter, not as a set of defective bronchial tubes that could maybe be fixed and maybe not. She gently pounded Mira's back to dislodge the mucus blocking her airway. She told us exactly what she was doing and showed us how to do it ourselves. And as she tended to Mira, she made gentle, practiced small talk that took my mind off the situation.

And she was right; it did look worse than it was. Mira's saturation level came up. She was admitted, but not intubated, and she recovered. Probably a dozen clinicians laid hands on Mira that day, but I remember—I will always remember—that nurse.

In February 2020, I was doing a bookstore event for my first book, *Early*, on the science and culture of premature birth, work inspired by Mira's early arrival. During a Q&A, one man told me his twins had been born quite prematurely—and then he said, "I just want you to talk about the NICU nurses. The NICU nurses meant so much to us." And then he started to cry.

I didn't know what to say because, frankly, thinking about the NICU nurses who cared for my daughter usually rendered me mute. I couldn't piece together an intelligent thought, but I remember saying something like "I loved them," and leaving it there. I had lived my way into a deep appreciation for nursing work—I knew that if you wanted something done, you had better ask a nurse (nicely)—but I had not yet taken the time to consider their role more deeply.

When I reflect more deliberately on the nurse who took care of Mira after her bronchoscopy, it becomes obvious how skilled and complex her practice was. At all times, she was working within several facets of nursing: She was handling the acute care Mira needed, watching her vital signs, adjusting the respiratory support accordingly, and consulting with the respiratory therapist. She was communicating with the rest of the health care team. When she explained how to dislodge the mucus blocking Mira's airways, an intervention known as chest PT, she was providing Mira with needed care and educating my husband and me at the same time. And by calming me—I'm sure it was obvious I needed calming—she was not simply being kind or humane, but was using an intervention that was also to Mira's benefit: research has shown that hospitalized kids may have better outcomes when their parents experience less anxiety.

By expressing both her skill and authority within the clinical situation and her compassion for me as a mother, that nurse built a trusting relationship with me in a matter of minutes. She made it comfortable for me to talk to her, and that was also a part of her expertise.

There's an oft-quoted observation that people may forget what you did, but they will never forget how you made them feel. This was true for me back then: what I remember most about that nurse is how she made me feel. But when we non-nurses focus on how nurses make us feel, we sometimes fail to recognize their knowledge, or we implicitly devalue their professionalism. We essentialize them in gendered ways: *She was like a mother, a sister.* We make saints or martyrs of them. We send them pizza or flowers while withholding the kind of respect and compensation physicians routinely command. In the long wake of the Covid-19 pandemic, perhaps many Americans have a better understanding of how much we all depend on nurses. But it's worth examining their place in our collective imagination and in our health care system and reckoning with how that affects the way they are treated, the ways they treat one another, the ways they are able to work—and, in turn, how that affects the kind of care available to all of us.

If I say "nurse," what do you think of? If you are a nurse, you might think of your work life and your colleagues and how you feel about the profession as a whole. If you're not, you might think of a nurse who helped you—or a time when a nurse couldn't or wouldn't help you. You might remember clapping for nurses during the early days of the pandemic. You might be reminded of being vulnerable, in need of care, and what that means to you. Perhaps, for you, a nurse is someone with frightening power over you; or you might think a nurse just follows doctors' orders. You might imagine Florence Nightingale, if she was the only nurse who you learned about at school. Maybe a feeling of comfort comes over you. Do you automatically think of a woman? Common stereotypes or caricatures might come to mind, like a "sexy nurse" Halloween costume. (An old vaudeville catcall is "Hello, Nurse!") Maybe Nurse Ratched from *One Flew Over the Cuckoo's Nest* pops into your head, or a character from *M*A*S*H* or *General Hospital* or *Misery*.

Many of the competing nurse stereotypes are misogynistic. While nursing is not an essentially female role, it has been gendered as such. These caricatures obscure the actual work of nursing and flatten the reality that nursing has many cultural meanings and involves some of the most intimate and profound interactions humans can have with one another. How we care for each other; how we wish to be cared for when we are sick, or injured, or in pain, or giving birth, or dying, or being born—these are some of the most highly charged experiences we have. Thinking about nursing work can be uncomfortable because it comes right up against our shared vulnerability.

Nursing is not just one practice; it represents an immense demographic. By some counts, it is the most populous profession in the world: There are more than 27 million professional nurses and midwives worldwide. Globally and in the United States, nurses constitute the largest group of health care professionals, and they provide most of the direct patient care. There are three times as many registered nurses in the United States as physicians. (Physicians are medical providers with an MD or a DO.) Health care would not be possible without nurses; the system simply could not function in their absence. Even nurses depend upon nurses.

There are many kinds of nurses, and the distinctions among them can be confusing. Nurses have both educational degrees and licenses. The degree tells you about their schooling; the license tells you that they passed an exam and are licensed to practice a particular kind of nursing with a certain scope. For instance, a BSN (bachelor of science in nursing) is a degree, while RN (registered nurse) refers to a license. You can be an RN with an associate's degree or a bachelor's degree. Regardless, every RN has passed the same licensing test, called the NCLEX-RN.

The American nursing workforce is made up of several groups, defined by licensure, education, or both: About sixty thousand nurses have doctorates; they do research, teach, work in policy, and practice clinically. There are about five hundred thousand advanced practice registered nurses (APRNs) in the United States. The nurses with this designation have at least a master's degree and specialty training and licensure; APRNs include nurse practitioners, clinical nurse specialists, nurse anesthetists, and nurse midwives. In most contexts, they can prescribe medication and provide independent health care, though, in about half of all states, they must work under physician "supervision." Registered nurses are the largest portion of the workforce; there are more than four million RNs in the United States; 90 percent are women, and 10 percent are men. About 80 percent identify as white, 6 percent as Hispanic/Latinx, 7 percent as Black, and 7 percent as Asian, of which Filipino nurses make up a significant portion. The RN workforce is disproportionately white compared to the population.

Other nurse licensures have different demographics and different educational requirements. Licensed practical nurses (LPNs) and licensed vocational nurses (LVNs) generally aren't required to have a college degree, though they must go through vocational training, and they must pass a licensing test. These practical nurses number about 940,000 and are more likely than RNs to be people of color. Certified nursing assistants (CNAs) number about 1.4 million; these professionals undergo a training program and then must pass a certification test. Many CNAs work in long-term care, like in skilled nursing facilities; women of color make up the majority of this workforce. The median annual salary for a CNA is $30,000, while the median annual salary for an RN is $77,000. These are all professional nursing categories.

More simply put, a present-day nurse is a trained and licensed health care professional who provides care for people in various settings, both acute (like hospitals) and non-acute (like schools, summer camps, nursing homes, and clinics). In fact, nurses are everywhere: On cruise ships, they manage stomach bug (or Covid-19) outbreaks. In libraries, they do free blood pressure checks. In church basements, they run diabetes support groups. In hospices, they manage pain. At NASA, they monitor astronauts. In birthing centers, they deliver babies. In legislatures, they write policy. In clinics and hospitals, they administer chemotherapy and renal dialysis, perform CPR, and provide patient education and support. They advocate for what is healthiest for the patient and community.

Everywhere, nurses notice and address problems before anyone else does. This could be a subtle change in a patient's mental status that presages a stroke, or a need for community-based vaccine education in a given area, or a pattern of kidney failure in agricultural workers during increasingly hot weather.

Nursing and medicine are two distinct but complementary and overlapping disciplines, and in theory at least, both nurses and physicians are there to use their respective skills to help the patient. Nurses do not work *for* physicians, but in concert with them. Medicine is one tool of nursing, but nursing is about more than procedures, medications, and cures.

Nurses manage patients' physiologies just as physicians do. (I'm thinking of that nurse monitoring my daughter's oxygen and managing her CPAP machine accordingly.) But physicians' practice generally goes deeper on the physiology (the intricate mechanisms of the body's biology), while nurses' practice is broader, including patient advocacy, preventative care, education, and the duty to assess and care for each patient holistically, as an individual in a given context—that is, within a family, a community, and an environment. In short, nurses integrate different kinds of information to understand the whole person.

If you are being discharged from a hospital, a nurse might ask: *Do you understand how to take your medication? Are there stairs to climb at home that you won't be able to manage? Are you on a special diet? Who does the cooking at home? Do you need food assistance?* If you're being discharged on supplemental oxygen: *Does anyone in the home smoke?* If you've been advised to take daily walks: *Do you feel safe in your neighborhood?* Ideally, a nurse problem-solves to maximize a patient's health and comfort, thinking beyond a given medication or remedy to how that patient lives in the world.

From a patient's point of view, sometimes it's not clear where one provider's job ends and another's begins—and this makes sense because ideally, the various providers will work as an interdisciplinary team. If, for instance, you need neurosurgery, a physician (a neurosurgeon) will perform the actual procedure, but it is nurses who will prep you for it: They'll insert the IV lines, check your vitals, and inventory the medications you're taking. Acting as a kind of air traffic control, it is nurses who will know how and when to pull in different disciplines: *Is a social worker needed? Has informed consent been given?*

During your surgery, an advanced practice nurse anesthetist or a physician anesthesiologist will administer the anesthesia and monitor your body's response. The surgical nurse will take part in the procedure, watching your overall condition. In the recovery room, the nurse anesthetist will ensure you come out of sedation as you should. The surgeon and her team will come check on you; write orders for medications, often in consultation with the nurse; and let you know how the surgery went. A nurse will administer those medications, watch your body's reaction to them, and adjust the meds accordingly. It is a nurse who will figure out when you can safely suck on ice chips and when to tell your family they can come see you. Incisions, IVs, medication management, skin health and infection control, instructions for at-home care—it is nurses who tend to all this in the aftermath of surgery, for you, your body, and your family. *Have you successfully used the bathroom post-surgery? Do you know what day it is? Is your pain being well managed? Does your family have unanswered questions?*

Nurses conceptualize their profession in a multitude of ways, but all emphasize how nursing is distinct from medicine. In her memoir, *Year of the Nurse*, Cassandra Alexander, RN, describes the difference between medicine and nursing like this: "They [doctors] learn where the patient *is* and demarcate where they want them to *be*. It is the bedside nursing that actually gets you there. Our hands are on the pumps and ventilators . . . Everything we do is an attempt to heal you."

Our hands are on the pumps and ventilators. This makes me think of when Mira was still in the NICU and stopped breathing. (This often happens with very premature babies; the complication is called apnea of prematurity.) Sometimes, the baby will start breathing again on her own; other times, a nurse will need to rub the infant's back or sternum to get her breathing. In this case, the nurse's gentle and then more vigorous rubbing did not make my daughter breathe. She was turning gray. So, the nurse reached with one hand for a bulb syringe and with the other for the bag and mask used to hand-resuscitate babies. With the syringe, she sucked mucus out of Mira's tiny nostril, and Mira drew in a shuddering breath and recovered. The episode was over—but when it began, that nurse did not stop to call a physician. She was ready to do whatever needed to be done. She made my daughter breathe with her own hands, and this was a completely routine part of her job.

Another part of a nurse's job is to advocate for the patient and to provide education and support for both the patient and their family.

In inpatient settings, nurses are there at the bedside—they don't come and go, as physicians do—so they are often able to build therapeutic relationships with patient families. This can be extremely complex work, requiring an ability to communicate compassionately and clearly in the most difficult situations.

"This is the difference between medicine and nursing," said Paula N. Kagan, PhD, RN, professor emerita at DePaul University. "Medicine is a cure discipline. It has a small repertoire of skills. I am not demeaning it. If you need brain surgery, if you need orthopedic surgery—you *need* that, and you want the best people to do it. But, then, who takes care of the person twenty-four/seven, after the surgeon goes in and does something for four hours? Physicians have a very narrow scope. They hate hearing this, but it's the truth. Ask any nurse. Nurses are the ones who heal the patients—actually, *help* heal, along with the person themselves and their family. Being in a mutual process with people, their families, and their communities—that's what nursing is."

When a nurse is in a mutual process with you, it might feel like simple kindness, like relief. But good nursing care is neither simple nor easy, though it might (it should) bring you ease and comfort. When the nurse let me wrap my arms around her while I was getting my emergency epidural, she was holding my body steady so that the anesthesiologist could position the catheter in my spine correctly. That is a routine nursing practice, but there is no way to fully describe what she was doing for me in quantifiable terms: her calmness in the midst of emergency; my arms around her still, solid body; steadying human contact at one of the scariest moments of my life. And the thing is, she might have been thinking about lunch—and that's fine.

The idea that the foundation of effective health care is the relationship between a patient and a nurse is a very old and archetypal one, but one way it was formalized and brought into modern hospital care was through the model of primary nursing, which emphasizes the therapeutic value in the connection between nurse and patient. The idea is that a patient should have the same primary nurse or nurses over the course of a hospitalization. This is an alternative to having an assortment of various nursing professionals provide fragmented care, with no one person fully responsible for the plan of care or the relationship. The model of primary care was co-developed by Marie Manthey, MNA, in 1969, and she came to it through personal experience: When she was five years old, she was quite ill and in the hospital. Her parents were allowed to visit only two times a week. "I felt abandoned, I felt anxious. I didn't know what was going to happen to me. I was afraid," Manthey said. "But one thing happened, and that is that a nurse, Florence Marie Fisher, sat down at my bedside. She colored in my coloring book, and that meant she cared for me. And I knew I wanted to be a nurse for the rest of my life." Fisher surely provided other aspects of health care for Manthey. But what Manthey remembered was the power of that relationship: Fisher seeing her and caring for her as a full human being. There is nothing woo-woo about that practice—it is profoundly effective in promoting well-being.

The idea of nursing as an identity rather than a job has often served to devalue nurses as scientific professionals, but many nurses do claim nursing as part of their identity. Monica McLemore, PhD, RN, a professor of nursing and public health at the University of Washington, said that being a nurse was fundamental to her worldview. And she sees the power of nursing as potentially transformative in people's lives.

"The magic of nursing really has to do with the fact that people don't understand the work that we actually, *really* do," McLemore said. "Nursing is not about skills and tasks. Yeah, we can put your IVs in with our eyes closed. But that's not the essence of nursing. The essence of nursing is we help families, individuals, and communities manage transitions. If that transition is from a disease state to a well state or from an injured state to a rehabilitation state—whatever that transition is, that's what we actually do. But everybody thinks it's skills and tasks. Reading a fetal heart monitor, being able to manage an intubated person—that's only one part; those are strategies for us to do our work. But our job is actually to get people back to some level of homeostasis, either back to where they started or better."

Many nurses have the sense that nursing should have a moral core, given how intimate nursing is with people's most vulnerable moments. In fact, the first qualification for RN licensure listed by the New York State Education Department is "good moral character." This feels very gendered in our time, but there has always been a concern that nurses behave ethically and not exploit their patients. In fact, this line of thinking goes all the way back to ancient India, when nurses were usually men. But in a modern professional context, who defines moral character?

Mark Lazenby, PhD, APRN, an oncology nurse and dean of the University of California, Irvine, Sue and Bill Gross School of Nursing, argues that the intimacy of nursing care is unique and integral to the profession in a way that has no comparison. Lazenby defines nursing's moral character as working through intimate care to create a better world for individuals and communities: "The moral character of nursing encompasses more than the feeling of caring. It involves caring in such a way that the better world is realized. . . . Nursing is a vocation with a profound morality built into its very nature."

Like most ideals, Lazenby's is not always realized. Nurses work in a pitiless system. We in the United States don't have a unified approach to maximizing people's health and well-being. We mostly have a for-profit medical industry focused on illness and conditions and, then, on potential billable cures and fixes. Health care workers generally do their very best to provide good care, but our "system" is often at cross-purposes with that effort. Nurses in particular, whose discipline is *not* medicine, are trying to work in a medical industry that was not built to make the most of their expertise or, really, even to recognize it. The fee-for-service model dictates that physicians—mainly the ones billing patients' insurance companies—are the revenue generators. Nursing is *just* as important to people's outcomes, but the fees for nursing are generally lumped in with hospital room and board—meaning that nursing is seen by hospitals as an expense, like meals or supplies. There are alternatives—like the successful single-payer socialized medical systems all over the world, where health care is seen as a human right. Within these other systems, nursing has the potential to be understood differently, because nurses excel at providing preventative care, health education, and interventions that lead to improved quality of life—which can make for a healthier population overall.

Teddie M. Potter, PhD, RN, of the University of Minnesota School of Nursing, said that our current medical system, with its rushed visits and lack of meaningful communication or connection, can result in patients and family members feeling confused, alienated, and unheard. Studies have shown that often physicians let patients speak for less than 30 seconds before they interrupt them. If there's a medication that might help, or a procedural fix, a physician is usually eager to provide it, but is not always able to listen long enough to understand all the patient's true needs. Potter acknowledges that, in this style of medical care delivery, a person's physical self can be treated effectively, and sometimes there's nothing more crucial than that. But other important aspects of ourselves and our health are lost; our minds, our spirits, our contexts, are often left behind. (*Severe, uncontrolled asthma. Lots of mucus and swelling. Bronchial tubes thirty percent smaller than expected!*—as that pulmonologist whizzes by.)

None of this is to denigrate physicians or medicine. Advances in medicine mean that millions of people have lived who, absent treatments for infections or prematurity or cancer—just to name three—would otherwise have died. But physicians, like nurses, are under pressure to work within a system that doesn't prioritize human connection, and their discipline is not inherently oriented toward such connection, though individual physicians certainly can be. Also, silos in medicine make it difficult to treat the whole person—literally. You might see a liver specialist, a neurologist, a gastroenterologist, and a psychiatrist, and each of them might carefully attend to their particular organ system, but good luck getting them to talk to one another or to you about the overall picture of your health.

The discipline of nursing can help fit those pieces back together and find ways to treat the full human being, which can improve outcomes in concrete ways. As Potter explained, "Our mind, body, spirit, we're all whole people . . . And [when you see your physician] you may feel like your needs are not being met. Yes, you may have received *responsible* care. It was not negligent. It wasn't malpractice. But it missed what you actually *need*. And so, it's seeing the whole person, over and over and over again. And that's what *nurses* do."

But nurses themselves do not always live up to their moral and ethical obligations to provide patient-centered care without bias. Nursing has its own serious internal problems, and those problems profoundly affect nurses' lives and their abilities to provide ethical care to the public. For instance, nursing has a very specific historical and present-day problem with racism. A 2021 study found that a staggering 92 percent of Black nurses say they have personally experienced racism directed against them in the workplace, from peer colleagues, nurse leaders, and patients in roughly equal numbers.

One way to start to tackle racism in nursing might be to make registered nursing less disproportionately white. And one way to do *that* might be to support the full inclusion of RNs with associate degrees (ADN), who are more likely to come from Black or brown or low-income communities. However, many hospitals are phasing out the hiring of registered nurses with associate degrees, even though those nurses pass the same licensing exam to become RNs as those with a bachelor's degree and are more likely to work in underserved areas that desperately need nurses. Patrick McMurray, MSN, RN, a nurse educator who teaches pharmacology to LPN and ADN-RN students at Robeson Community College in North Carolina, says that restricting the profession to those who can access a bachelor's program and not supporting community college pathways to nursing are clearly disproportionate bars to groups that have already been excluded from registered nursing—Black and brown people, first-generation college students, immigrants, and low-income people. This issue is reflective of the ways racism and classism complicate nursing, and these tensions are very old.

Nursing often operates from a harmful sense of scarcity: Many hospitals do not hire enough nurses to meet the needs of the community, and there are constant nurse staffing shortages in the United States. This is not a simple *nurse* shortage per se—although, in some contexts, more nurses are needed—but a long-standing crisis in staffing brought about by poor working conditions. Nursing has high turnover, which is directly related to unsafe working conditions and the moral distress that arises from that. A new national survey found that nurses face inadequate staffing levels, a lack of personal protective equipment, mental health challenges, and even workplace violence. Sixty-two percent of nurses reported being verbally abused at work. From within and without, nursing is tightly bound into power dynamics of gender, race, and class. It is associated with female domestic labor, with the nurse cast as a submissive helpmeet but expected to perform miracles. Many nurses end up feeling thwarted in their original desire to help people.

Historian Susan M. Reverby, PhD, investigated this dynamic

in her seminal book on nursing, *Ordered to Care*: "As some nursing moved out of the realm of unpaid family labor into the marketplace, the assumption that it would still be work of love, not money, remained. The ideology of nursing, based on nineteenth-century understandings of women's duties, but not of women's rights, gave trained nursing purpose but limited its power to control or define its occupational or professional existence." This ideology lingers today.

Julie Jenkins, DNP, APRN, often finds herself intensely frustrated by nursing as it is, and she fights for nursing as it could be: "A phrase that we say is 'Nurses eat their young.' No one's saying it's a good thing, but it's *just what happens*—instead of [our] saying, 'Hey, why have we ever *let* this happen? We need to change this.'" Some nurses, like Jenkins and others who have lent their stories to this book, *are* changing it, constructing ways of nursing that are both new and very, very old.

Nursing is, and has always been, both uncommonly complicated and uncommonly powerful. In considering nursing of the past and present, there are irreconcilable tensions in how nursing is defined—as a biological science and as hands-on caring, as professional and as domestic, as skills and as relationships, as knowing in the mind and knowing in the body. I think all these can be true and that those complications are part of nursing's power.

This book is a love letter to nursing's vast possibilities. I have been on the receiving end of nursing care so expert and compassionate that it altered my life. I know that this kind of care is possible and that it should be possible for all of us. So, my purpose here is not to represent *all* of nursing—that would be impossible—but to argue for the inherent power of ethical nursing to recognize and address problems, to create a better and more just world, and to alleviate suffering. I want both nurses and non-nurses to understand that nurses have changed the world and continue to do so.

The strengths of nursing, when traced from the past into the present, have deep and urgent relevance to the problems confronting us right now. We are facing an escalating crisis of caring, in many domains. Even problems outside the obvious realm of health care—climate change, policy leadership, the built environment, loss of community—have huge impacts on human health. Nurses see the symptoms of these problems written on their patients' bodies. As we face these interrelated crises—which all come back to the absolute urgency of caring for one another—all of us need to understand nursing's power to see and to act. Many of the nurses in this book are using their unique insight to tackle today's problems. We ignore their expertise at our own peril.

What if we all recognized how false hierarchies have suppressed nursing knowledge, only making it harder for us to get the care we need? What if telling different stories about nursing changed the way our society valued nursing expertise? And what would it look like if more great nurses used their hard-won insights to lead—if they had the budgets, the authority, the safety to do that work? A world like that might be a more caring, healthier place for everyone.

CHAPTER 1

ORIGINS

To Nurse Is to Be Human:
Reclaiming a History

*No matter whether this treatment is carried out
by sorcerers, priests, doctors, or old women, we
find examples of the historic ancestry of modern
nursing and the earliest forms of the art.*

—LAVINIA L. DOCK, RN, AND MARY ADELAIDE
NUTTING, RN, *A HISTORY OF NURSING*

Nursing is a thread running through all human history: Nurses were at the events that defined our world. They were key to the success of the Byzantine and Roman and Indian Empires. They were instrumental in the founding of the world's major religions. They were tried as witches; they were forced underground—but they never stopped passing down what they knew, even when it was dangerous. They were arrested for providing birth control and jailed for trying to vote. They acted on their expertise even when enslaved; they broke down Jim Crow. They went where they were needed, and they fought for everyone's right to a good death. They brought their knowledge to the halls of government. Human societies simply could not have developed and functioned the way that they have without nursing.

So, if you imagine that nursing arose only in relatively recent times, as a profession dedicated to assisting physicians within hospitals, you have it backward. Nursing came first.

Historians and anthropologists often point to pivotal moments that distinguished the evolution of early humans: when we started making tools or decorative objects, or using fire to cook, or when we cooperated by sharing food. But what about the impulse to staunch someone's bleeding? What about helping someone give birth? What about sitting up with someone who was dying? These are interactions that define humans as much as the use of tools, fire, and agriculture.

Four thousand years ago, in a Neolithic Stone Age community in what is now Bach Lien Village, Vietnam, a baby boy was born with Klippel-Feil syndrome, a rare congenital condition in which neck vertebrae are fused together. As he grew, the boy curled. His spinal column became progressively compressed, until he was paralyzed from the waist down, with very little use of his upper body. His head twisted to the right; he could not feed himself. Chewing and swallowing were probably difficult. Nevertheless, even after becoming almost completely immobile as a teenager, he lived until his mid-twenties. Someone, or many someones, must have nursed him intensively. They brought him food and water, fed him, bathed him. They would have had to help him with positioning and tend to his skin, to prevent pressure sores and infections. Without nursing care, he would have died within days.

When the young man died, he was buried in the fetal position, because of the curve in his spine. When archeologists found him in 2007, they noticed that he was the only one in the community buried in this way. Then they saw the fused neck vertebrae, and the extreme slenderness of his leg and arm bones that comes with paralysis. Lorna Tilley, PhD, an archeologist on the dig, had previously worked in nursing. The young man's body spoke to her, and she started to piece this case together with other evidence of prehistoric nursing.

In the 1980s, archeologists uncovered an eight-thousand-year-old peat bog burial ground in Florida. Among the bodies was that of a sixteen-year-old boy who had survived since birth with disabling spina bifida. The skeleton of a young woman was discovered at a Bronze Age site near what is now Dubai. Her bones indicated that she had suffered from polio, which left her paralyzed from the waist down. The muscle markers on the bones of her upper body suggested that she used her arms to drag herself around. She would have needed nursing to survive the severe viral stage of the illness and then would have required assistance for the rest of her life.

Tilley became captivated by what these bones were saying, but when she looked back at previous archeological studies, she found that while survival from illness or injury was sometimes noted, there was often little to no analysis or even acknowledgment of the prehistoric nursing care that would have made this survival possible. Informed by her work in both archaeology and health care, she developed a model called the bioarcheology of care, a framework for understanding how our earliest ancestors nursed one another.

In *Anthropology News*, Tilley and her coauthor, Alecia Schrenk, argued for the importance of understanding ourselves this way: "Our past contains important lessons for our present if we are willing to pay attention," they wrote. "An archeological focus on health-related care completely overturns the notion that society has evolved by embracing a winner-takes-all, 'survival of the fittest' approach to health and welfare policy. . . . A defining hallmark of the human species is our capacity to support each other in times of need."

Of course, modern professional nursing, with its scientific knowledge and evidence-based practices, is very different from ancient nursing. But modern nursing's origins—the organized impetus behind it—can be traced all the way back to the skilled hands that tended to that paralyzed boy. Even when nursing is elided in general history books and archeology studies, it is still there. You can see it sometimes only in outline, in relief: in every heroic tale of survival, there is an invisible hand that stopped the bleeding. Can we be human *without* nursing?

The voices of those doing the nursing are not often in the dominant historical narratives—perhaps because the caregivers were often women or enslaved people, or were otherwise subordinated; or, perhaps, because caring work has frequently been domestic, not done in public, obscured by its own private ordinariness; or, perhaps, because those writing the histories were more interested in tales of domination, empire building, and violence than of partnership and healing. When healing is addressed, it is often credited to physicians, who are positioned as some of the "great men" of history, even though nurses have always played an indispensable role in restoring a person to health, often the major role.

Nurses themselves have long wondered at this silence about what came before, and nursing historians have painstakingly excavated stories that were originally neglected.

In 1907, two American nurses, Mary Adelaide Nutting, RN, and Lavinia L. Dock, RN, wrote a sprawling four-volume world history of nursing for nurses. It chronicled care from ancient Babylon and India through medieval and early modern Europe. "In attempting to study the history of nursing, which must always have existed in some form, however rude, we find long ages of silence on the subject, doubtless because of this tendency of historians to overlook what is usual and homely," they write. Their writing was an attempt to correct the record and to connect the nurses of their day with the long line of knowledge that stretched out behind them—to give both inspiration and perspective, not just because it would be nice to know, but because it would change the way nurses understood their own potential.

More than one hundred years later, nurses and nursing historians have continued these efforts to illuminate. Writing in 2019 about the long history of nursing in Egypt, nurses Sameh Elhabashy and Elshaimaa M. Abdelgawad echoed Nutting and Dock's line of thinking. They argued that present-day nurses needed a historical framework to develop their own professional identity. "Nursing has a long and rich history, yet this is rarely conveyed to current nursing students, which makes them devalue the achievements of earlier nurses," they write.

You might be surprised to hear that nursing goes back to Neolithic times, that it is a fundamental human impulse that has found skilled expression in many times and places—and you'd be excused for not knowing this because just about every mainstream source, from the History Channel to Wikipedia, cites Florence Nightingale, an upper-class lady of Victorian England, as the sole founder of modern nursing. But, like most lone-hero narratives, this one is not entirely true. Nightingale herself trained with a venerable group of German deaconess nurses. She did advocate for nursing as a trained profession and for public health sanitation measures, but as she did so, she shrank nursing into a restrictive, exclusionary Victorian corset, constructing a version of nursing that conformed to rigid social mores, one divided by class, race, and gender. The absolute focus on Nightingale as *the* prototypical nurse has stripped nursing of its truer, more sweeping history and of the power that lies within that.

Nursing did not spring fully formed out of Nightingale's England. And the Victorian idea that modern nursing is a profession for well-off white women, and mostly for the purposes of ensuring hygiene and carrying out physicians' orders, is not only misleadingly narrow, but also harmful. When nursing is so small in the collective imagination, we all lose out on its potential for making a better world.

What follows is a brief, not-at-all comprehensive journey back through time and place to illuminate nursing's many origins. Where did nursing come from? It came from everywhere. How could it be otherwise? All people in all places and in all times have lived in these beautiful, transient, vulnerable human bodies.

Domestic nursing was likely the first kind of skilled care: done in the home, usually by family or community experts. Historian Leigh Whaley, PhD, proposes that all health care grew out of the home, "practiced by mothers and handed down through the ages by their mothers, grandmothers and great-grandmothers." The word *nurse* comes from the Latin verb for "nourish," a word with many meanings. But ancient nursing took place outside the home, too—in religious traditions, at war, and in the establishment of collective health infrastructure, like home nursing services, hospitals, hospices, and pharmacies. Nursing has been fundamental to establishing human societies and cultures.

We can follow these threads back more than two thousand years to ancient India, where ayurveda, the traditional medicine of Hinduism, placed deep cultural and practical importance on the role of the nurse. The Charaka-Samhita, one of ayurveda's major texts, states that there are four fundamental pillars of health care: the patient, the nurse, the physician, and the medicine. All four have different but critical roles; without any one of them, health care would not exist. That text also sets forth qualifications for health care professionals. It specifies that both physicians and nurses should have knowledge about dosing and administering medicines, but it emphasizes scriptural education for physicians, while hands-on skill and sterling character would qualify nurses.

Dock and Nutting quote an ancient Indian text that argues that nurses should be "of good behavior, distinguished for purity, possessed of cleverness and skill, imbued with kindness, skilled in every service a patient may require, competent to cook food, skilled in bathing and washing the patient, rubbing and massaging the limbs, lifting and assisting him to walk about, well skilled in making and cleansing of beds, readying the patient and skillful in waiting upon one that is ailing." It is a comprehensive description, and one not entirely unfamiliar in our own world.

Not only was there a cultural-religious framework for the nurse's role, but as always, there was also a pragmatic need for nurses as health care infrastructure was built—and health care infrastructure was *big* in ancient India, a fact often credited to Buddhist emperor Ashoka, who came to power around 270 BCE. (Buddhism grew out of Hinduism and shares many texts and practices with it, including ayurveda.) In paintings and sculpture, Ashoka is mustachioed and fit, with a cleft chin, gold hoop earrings, and flowing black hair. His focus on health care came as a kind of redemption project, after he unleashed terrible bloodshed in expanding his empire. The story goes that he was so guilt-ridden by the carnage that he renounced violence and dedicated himself to dharma, the pursuit of righteousness.

Ashoka's dharmic redemption required nurses, as he ordered that a sophisticated hospital network be built throughout the subcontinent, where both physicians and nurses tended to patients and compounded medicines. He also built training programs and, around 250 BCE, established a formal nursing school—likely the first in the world. In the hospitals, the nurses (usually men) would have provided care based on ayurvedic principles, including dosing medication, helping patients bathe and eat, and providing massage. Patient happiness and overall mood were considered integral to health: Hospitals were encouraged to have musicians on hand, and artists who could recite legends. As Buddhism and its practices spread to Sri Lanka, so did this system of hospital care and the trained nursing that made it possible.

Or, we can follow those threads even farther back in time, to ancient Egypt, 3,500 years ago, where nurses and physicians, who were often priests, enjoyed special status because health was explicitly tied to the relationship between humans and the gods. A person could stay healthy by keeping the gods happy; if you got sick, physicians and nurses would treat both your physical symptoms and what they understood as the supernatural cause. Nurses were both men and women, but the two sexes seemed to have different roles. Working alongside physicians, male nurses provided supportive care during illness, such as positioning patients, feeding them, and monitoring temperature and pulse. Midwives, for their part, were exclusively women, and their work seems to have been especially linked with the divine, as they are depicted as goddesses in birthing scenes. Other nurses cared for children, often as wet-nurses, but also in other ways, like tutoring and keeping children safe and healthy. The distinctions among different kinds of care were not like our own. Royals had their own private nurses, who were always close by. Queen Hatshepsut's nurse, Sitre, was buried side by side with the queen, despite not being from a royal family, a sign of her importance and the intimacy of their relationship.

Zipping forward in time to ancient Rome, we arrive at around 100 CE: There, while most health care for citizens occurred privately, in homes, hospitals with nursing care were built for the military as a way of protecting the sprawling empire. It's very hard to win wars and maintain control without nurses to care for the armed forces; fortunes and empires can rise and fall on their work.

Roman military hospitals, called *valetudinaria*, were large, airy buildings with operating rooms, baths, and shrines to Hygeia, the Roman goddess of health. The facilities could accommodate up to five hundred patients at a time and were dotted throughout the empire, usually near military forts and camps. There, soldiers and sailors received care not just for war wounds, but also for ailments common to living in close quarters and traveling: respiratory viruses, sexually transmitted infections, food poisoning, injuries from accidents. One account, from 115 CE, tells of a young soldier who had to go to a *valetudinarium* for "fish poisoning."

Medici, or physicians, which included surgeons, were on staff, but the routine care was often provided by *capsarii* (named after the capsa, a box containing bandages), or what we might call nurses. All the health care workers were men. The care at the time was based on the ancient Greek theory of the four humors, which held that the body has four fundamental substances: blood, phlegm, black bile, and yellow bile. Any illness was thought to be caused by an imbalance in those substances, which often meant you needed to get rid of a surplus of one of them. This is why purging by bleeding, emetics, diuretics, laxatives, and the draining of pus was considered a legitimate medical treatment. So, nurses doled out substances that would make a patient vomit, or they would nick a vein to let it bleed, or lance a boil to release pus. The humors theory was accepted throughout the West for more than two thousand years, and many nursing practices revolved around it.

But *capsarii* also provided basic infection control and comfort care, which was probably somewhat effective even when the bleedings and laxatives were not: *capsarii* used vinegar to wash wounds, honey to prevent infection, turmeric to lessen inflammation. They administered first aid, which included the use of tourniquets, and administered opium for pain or, if surgery was needed, a combination of opium and wine to create a kind of anesthesia. When true medical cures were few and far between, supportive nursing care was key to any possible healing.

From ancient Rome, fast-forward five hundred years to what is now Saudi Arabia, for a particularly potent story that combines the threads of religion and war: a nurse was instrumental in the 7th century birth of Islam. Rufaida Al-Aslamiya grew up watching her father, a health practitioner, care for their neighbors in Medina. As she got older, she apprenticed with him and learned what he knew: first aid, medicines for fever, ways to prevent infection. Then in 622 CE, a man named Muhammad came to their town calling himself the Prophet of Allah, the one true god. He had been driven out of his hometown, Mecca, where most were polytheists and where Muhammad's new, monotheistic religion threatened the status quo. Rufaida heard him speak about how the angel Jibreel had appeared to him with revelations, and she became a believer. As Muhammad's reputation grew, his conflict with the polytheistic Meccans grew also, until Muhammad embarked on a series of battles to bring the region under his control.

The human toll was horrific—as it always is in war, but especially when there's no one to take care of the casualties. Rufaida realized that her skills could mitigate the suffering. She recruited and trained a group of women to travel with Muhammad's army and provide care—first aid for wounds, comfort for the dying. To shield the injured from the harsh sun and wind, her team of nurses erected tents for field hospitals in the desert; they kept bedding and wounds clean and provided drinking water and food. One account describes how Rufaida was able to remove an arrow from the arm of one of Muhammad's closest companions, stopping him from bleeding to death. The care she provided was so essential to the outcome of the war that Muhammad ordered that she be paid the same share of spoils as his soldiers.

After Muhammad gained control of Mecca, he asked Rufaida to put up a tent on the grounds of his Nabawi mosque in Medina to provide primary care and health education; it was a position of authority, so it is clear that he highly valued Rufaida's expertise. She practiced broadly, championing preventative care and education—a distinctly nursing perspective. Omar Hasan Kasule, MD, a professor of epidemiology who has studied Rufaida, wrote, "She did not confine her nursing to the clinical situation. She went out to the community and tried to solve the social problems that lead to disease."

Public health care subsequently became very important in the early Islamic world. One thousand years ago—and five hundred years after Rufaida—there were dozens of sophisticated hospitals, called *bimaristans*, in Iraq, Iran, Syria, Egypt, Saudi Arabia, and Tunisia. In Baghdad alone, there were at least six. Skilled nursing was key to the care provided there. Many bimaristans had their own pharmacy and library and were what we now call teaching hospitals, where knowledge was shared and built upon. When a patient was ready to go home, they received a bath, a new set of clothes, and some money to get back on their feet. It was an acknowledgment of the many costs of being ill, and a precursor to nursing discharge planning.

Around that same time, in Constantinople (now Istanbul), a nurse, who also happened to be a historian, was tending to her dying father, who also happened to be the emperor. Her account is a rare first-person narrative from a nurse of the time and a glimpse into in-home care.

Anna Komnene was the daughter of Alexius I, who ruled the Byzantine Empire from 1081 until his death in 1118. During Anna's time, the empire encompassed all of what is now Turkey and Greece and some of southeastern Europe. Anna was an avid reader, highly educated, and she is most remembered for writing a fifteen-volume history of her father's reign, *The Alexiad*. But she was also a knowledgeable and skilled nurse who tried to save her father's life.

In *The Alexiad*, Anna recalls how she first overheard her parents talking worriedly about her father's symptoms. "And I often heard him speaking about it to my mother . . . 'What in the world is this disease which has attacked my breathing? For I should like to take a deep, full breath and get rid of this trouble worrying my heart.'" As her father struggled to breathe, a worried Anna took charge of his care. She consulted with many of the prominent physicians of Constantinople, taking some of their advice, but disregarding some, too. She brought in physicians to bleed her father, but it had no effect. They tried pepper as a purgative, and he improved for a day but then declined again. He could breathe only while sitting up; while lying down, he gasped. When he finally fell asleep, Anna feared he would suffocate. "For not even a moment could he draw breath freely," she writes. Her mother took to sitting up all night with him, holding him upright in her arms. She and Anna changed his bedclothes, experimented with his positioning. It might seem strange that Anna and her mother, royals themselves, were doing all this, rather than hired nurses, but while Anna accepted advice from others, she felt qualified and clearly wanted to care for her father herself.

The emperor's abdomen became distended, his feet bloated; his tongue swelled in his mouth. Physicians arrived at Anna's direction to apply cauterization, in which skin is burned with hot metal, a practice thought to have therapeutic effect. It didn't. The emperor stopped eating. Anna prepared his food herself, making dishes that were easy to swallow. "All things pointed to the end," she writes. When it came, she kept her hand on her father's pulse. "I touched it again and I recognized that all his strength was giving way and that the pulse in the arteries had finally stopped, then I bowed my head and, exhausted and fainting, I looked down to the ground, said nothing, but clasped my hands over my face and stepped back and wept."

Imagine, through millennia, so many like her: Nurses who were not the emperor's daughter and, so, did not leave written accounts, but who also stood at a bedside and felt a pulse as it faded away. Anna was acting across several nursing identities: she had her own knowledge and consulted with other experts as she made her plan of care. Throughout her life, she would provide health care for people both inside and outside her family. She treated her husband's tumor and wrote about the possible causes for it. She diagnosed a Norman duke with fever and pleurisy. For her father, she acted as a family caregiver, perhaps the oldest kind of nurse.

Anna's account is precious because nursing done in homes (even castles) was more likely to be performed by women and to be unrecorded. Historian Monica H. Green has shown that only a fraction of medieval female practitioners was ever officially counted. This has a present-day corollary: If you came back from the future and wanted to try to figure out how our medical system worked, you might logically start with the medical journals of today. You'd probably surmise that *most* health care was provided by physicians—particularly male physicians—because that's who is published most often. Or you might read newspaper articles about health care in which physicians were most often the cited experts. You might not understand just from reading what is published in mainstream sources that today's health care runs on nursing.

After Anna's father died, her brother, John II, became the new Byzantine emperor, and with him, we can pick up a different thread: medieval Byzantine health care infrastructure, which was incredibly sophisticated, depended on a robust professional nursing workforce. John II, who would become known as John the Good, built the Pantokrator, one of the most advanced hospitals of the time.

In its heyday one thousand years ago, the Pantokrator had sprawling grounds, an organized system of rounds, and a plan of care for each patient. There were fifty inpatient beds, divided into specialty wards—for example, one for epilepsy, one for eye problems, and one just for women. There was also an outpatient clinic, a pharmacy, baths, and a bakery with a mill for grinding flour. (Byzantine hospital food involved wine, warm bread, and vegetables cooked in olive oil.) Some of the complex still stands today, an imposing, big-shouldered building made of pinkish stone, now known as the Zeyrek Mosque. The very existence of the Pantokrator vividly contradicts the idea that organized nursing care originated in nineteenth-century Western Europe.

About twenty licensed physicians rotated in and out of the hospital in short-term residencies, but the large nursing staff of about forty-six was permanent, made up of professionals who had passed a licensing test to qualify for the job. The nursing schedule was organized into two shifts of twelve hours a day, as is common now. Nurses were men who cared for men (*hypourgoi*) and women who cared for women (*hypourgisses*), and the two sexes earned the same wage.

There are clues to the daily life of Pantokrator hospital nurses in stories like this one: In 1140, Theodoros Prodromos, royal poet at John the Good's court, broke out in a fever and a pustulant rash. Historian Guenter B. Risse, PhD, uncovered what Prodromos wrote to a friend: "God hit me with a painful sore through the whole body . . . I have now been thrown into the most disgraceful condition to look at and suffer pestilence." Prodromos even wrote a poem about how terrible he felt: "The forest's mist sends a chill through my brain, colder than the sacred grove of olives and rain comes down from the mountain clouds." He may have had smallpox, a deadly and common disease at the time.

The poet was admitted to the Pantokrator. There, in consultation with physicians, the nurses would have provided care designed to bring his body back into humoral balance. The erupting smallpox sores leaked pus and were considered an example of the body's natural purging. Treatments were aimed at speeding that process along: Prodromos may have been put in a steam room to sweat; then, nurses would have rubbed him all over with cloths to wipe away the sweat and pus. They would have bathed him, massaged him, and bled him. He submitted to cauterization very unwillingly, with nurses holding him down while a physician performed the procedure. Prodromos was eventually well enough to leave the hospital and lived for another sixteen years.

We are lingering here in the Middle Ages, the thousand-year span of 500 to 1500 CE, because it was a dynamic time for the development of organized health care and for the expansion of nursing care around the world. In Western Europe—at the same time that *bimaristans* flourished in the Middle East and North Africa, and as Prodromos was being admitted to the Pantokrator in Constantinople—nursing was becoming increasingly organized around the Christian idea of faith through works and charity. Phoebe, a deaconess in the New Testament, is often cited as a model of an early nurse who cared for the poor and sick. As Christianity spread, many nuns and monks took up the work of nursing. And throughout the European Middle Ages, it was often religious communities that established the first hospices, clinics, pharmacies, and hospitals.

Monasteries and convents lent themselves to the provision of health care. For one thing, they often had facilities (like large halls) that could serve as clinics or pharmacies; they also had libraries, gardens in which to grow medicinal herbs, and kitchens in which to compound those herbs into medicines. And they often had an infirmary for their own members as they aged or grew ill, care that could then be expanded outward to serve the wider community.

Some of the first public health care in Europe would not have been possible without nursing nuns. The Augustinian Sisters of Paris, one of the oldest nursing orders, provided care at Paris's Hôtel Dieu hospital starting in 651 and continuing for an astonishing twelve hundred years. (The Hôtel Dieu is still in operation.) The sisters lived at the hospital for life, their nursing considered a manifestation of their having dedicated their lives to god and to the ideal of care for impoverished people. Versions of this arrangement were relatively common: the Franciscan Hospitallers of France, Belgium, and the Netherlands were nursing sisters who, in the fourteenth century, established many of their own hospitals and also visited people at home to care for them.

The Middle Ages was not generally a time of great health. The deadliest outbreak of disease ever recorded was the Black Death plague of the 1300s, and waves of infectious disease rippled across Europe and Asia throughout the Middle Ages and Renaissance. In that context, nursing was often a radically compassionate act of bravery in the face of death. Many nuns and monks died while nursing others through outbreaks of plague—a refusal to let people die alone and uncomforted that has echoes in our own time. Amid the Black Death, a small hospital next to Thornton Abbey in Lincolnshire, England, took in dozens of people from the surrounding community, all of them infected with the plague. In 2013, workers excavated a mass grave on the site, uncovering the remains of forty-eight men, women, and children who had died during that epidemic, each of them carefully shrouded and buried nestled together.

Even in less fraught moments, nuns and monks provided crucial care. In her book *Acts of Care*, historian Sara Ritchey, PhD, describes the work of religious women in the late Middle Ages in what is now the Netherlands and Belgium: "Women living as beguines and Cistercian nuns in this region served as nurses, herbalists, everyday caretakers, and wonder-workers who assisted patients using charms, blessings, relics, meditations, and prayers, in addition to herbs, stones, purgatives, phlebotomy, and maintenance of a daily regimen."

One particularly vibrant example of this everyday caretaking, this "wonder-work," brings us forward in time, out of the Middle Ages and into the Renaissance, to the elaborate apothecaries built by the nuns of Florence, Italy, starting in the 1500s. There, nuns sold remedies and wellness products and offered health advice and religious comfort. These early pharmacies were appealing community spaces where women came for help on health matters of all kinds.

The popular apothecary of the Santa Caterina nuns, for instance, was an inherently social place, where well-off ladies came to shop for perfumes, wellness products, and medicines, while less-well-off women of the neighborhood would have come in for an urgent remedy. The shop would have been full of heady fragrances and lined with carefully labeled jars filled with herbs, tinctures, and distillates. (Many convents used medicinal herbs and flowers from their own gardens, but they also traded with the wider world for needed items.) Historian Sharon T. Strocchia, PhD, vividly describes the scene at the Santa Caterina apothecary in her book *Forgotten Healers*:

Among the jars and vials there was sorrel distillate for fever, especially sought after because malaria was endemic in Tuscany at that time. There was also essence of violet and rose, mixed into ointments and medicinal oils, and distillates of betony, an all-purpose herbal remedy for digestive and respiratory illnesses. Rhubarb (also a mainstay of Chinese medicine) was boiled into syrups or distillates, to be used as a laxative. There were brandies. There was soap, which was just becoming popular as people started to associate cleanliness with good health and status, and other goods, like perfumes and ointments, that we might think of as wellness products. The nuns even sold rich chicken broth for convalescents. And, of course, there was also a religious element to their nursing practice. For instance, the nuns might give a woman a blessed amulet to wear around her neck for fertility.

Ultimately, the nursing work of religious women was often recorded as acts of godliness and purity, but not of knowledge or training. Historian Ritchey makes this point through the story of a young beguine. (Beguines were religious communities of unmarried women who were not nuns.) This particular beguine was named Ida, and she was called to the home of a man who was nearly dead from an illness that involved a pus-filled abscess. Ida ably drained the pus, and the man recovered. But instead of noting her nursing skill, the monk who recorded her story immortalized it as an act of virginal holiness. As Ritchey writes, "Her therapeutic actions were recorded not as demonstrations of medical acumen but as examples of her intense religiosity."

This is just one example of nursing skill being written out of history. There is a misconception that nuns who nursed were *just* religious, that they were not doing much at all except praying; perhaps providing spiritual comfort, maybe a miracle or two. On the contrary, nursing has always been nothing if not practical and hands-on. Credibility and evidence were important for early nurses, even those mostly outside the scholarly world. In letters to their clients, for instance, nun apothecaries often included reassuring "proofs," citing examples of how many times this herb or concoction had been shown to be effective. Religion has provided an infrastructure for nursing and internal motivation for some of those who did the work—whether the nurses were inspired by Muhammad, the Charaka-Samhita, or the Bible—but many of these religious people were, in fact, doing the very practical, human-centered work of nursing, which was not just thoughts and prayers.

Finally, one last jump forward in time—this time, to the United States starting around 1619 and during the following 246 years of slavery: Here, enslaved people carried and passed down nursing and midwifery practices grounded in their spiritual beliefs. This legacy is very much alive in American nursing today, even when it is not properly credited or understood.

Kidnapped from different parts of the African continent and from various cultures, enslaved people brought their knowledge and practices with them; some even managed to carry seeds for medicinal plants, like okra, woven into their hair. Once here, they integrated many of these traditions into distinctly African American practices of folk medicine, some aspects of which are called Hoodoo or conjure. Religious scholar Stephanie Y. Mitchem, PhD, defines African American folk healing in this way: "In this view, human life is understood relationally as part of the interconnected, shared web of the universe. Sickness, then, is derived not only from germs but also from situations that break relational connections." This view was carried by many African American people into their nursing and midwifery work.

Enslaved people practiced nursing care freely in their own communities and as enslaved labor in both Black and white communities. In fact, they provided most of the nursing in the slave states. Midwives delivered babies of all races. Older enslaved women who could no longer work the fields were often forced to nurse in infirmary houses, caring for fellow enslaved people. Or, an enslaved woman might be ordered to tend to a white family's sick child, only to find herself accused of poisoning the child if they died.

But enslaved nurses and midwives also *chose* to provide care. Elder women were often revered for their health knowledge. There was resistance in the act of sitting up with the sick, in making sure they had a good place by the fire, something to eat. There was resistance in midwives' provision of contraceptive and abortion care when it was prohibited, as enslaved women's reproduction was a matter of financial gain for enslavers. These nurses knew how to use the pharmacopeia of the natural world: They soaked pine needles in very hot water and used the vapor to cure a cough. They prescribed cotton root for contraception. They administered teas and tinctures. They used herbs and roots for fever and infection. They delivered babies and washed the dead. Sociologist Dorothy Roberts, PhD, cautions against romanticizing this kind of work, noting that enslaved women had to work a gendered double duty: in the field or house as slave labor *and* in their own communities. Nevertheless, as Roberts also points out, it's equally important to understand these practices as a font of skill that benefited African American communities.

Nursing as resistance took particularly spectacular form in the life of Jane Minor, also called Jensey (or Gensey) Snow. Minor was set free in 1825 for what her enslaver called "extraordinary merit in nursing" during a fever epidemic. As a free woman, she opened a hospital in Petersburg, Virginia, where she worked for more than thirty years. With the money she earned providing care, she purchased the freedom of sixteen enslaved people, including mothers with children, and at least one other nurse.

African American folk medicine practices, and that relational view of health, are specific to African American communities and, in fact, were suppressed, derided, and stolen by white people. Nevertheless, these practices, and the relational way of looking at health, went where African American nurses went and have become a hallmark of nursing—indeed, they are part of what distinguishes nursing from other health care disciplines.

These stories are a tiny fraction of the myriad ways nurses have worked across time and place and of the many meanings of nursing care. There is no one origin story for nursing; there are uncountable origin stories, and that multiplicity argues that nursing is fundamental to human life.

Nurses have driven history in ways that have often been rendered invisible. Nursing has been practical and everyday. Nursing has been extraordinary acts of bravery. Nursing has been a conviction that everyone deserves comfort. Nursing has been knowledge and expertise in action. The history of nursing argues that nursing belongs to everyone.

CHAPTER 2

HIERARCHY

The Making of a Big Lie: Essentially Female, Always Subordinate

If nursing can be traced to Neolithic times and ancient empires—if it was performed by men and women, mothers and daughters, soldiers and enslaved people, and monks and nuns and priestesses who wielded their skill and authority to bring comfort and healing—how did we arrive here, at a time when much of the public and many nurses don't know these stories or their meanings?

Most of the general public understands nursing as a set of tasks, like handing out medication, and taking blood pressure, likely performed by a female nurse at the behest of a physician. Medication and vital sign management are very important ways of taking care of people, but they are only a fraction of nursing's scope. Also, there is a pervasive view that nursing is somehow "naturally" done by women, even though the past and present contradict this. There is nothing inherently wrong with an association with feminine, or maternal, care, but the idea that nursing is, by definition, a female practice has not been good for anyone. And among non-nurses, there is a limited understanding of nursing as an independent discipline, one not defined in relation to physicians, but instead as a science that is continually advanced by the ongoing work of nurse scholars. So, how did nursing come to be so poorly understood as essentially female labor that is subordinate to physicians?

The short answer is that, in the European and North American context, the idea of modern nursing was built to fit into a modern medical hierarchy, one that put university-educated physicians at the top and deliberately squashed every other kind of expert caring. As a discipline, nursing got pruned into a shape that could accommodate this new story, the one that says physicians are the only heroes and that everyone else is only a supporting character.

Here is the longer answer: In the European Middle Ages, the health care landscape was more fluid than our own, but it had a certain logic: If you had a stomachache or a fever, you might go to a local convent or monastery, where nuns and monks sold remedies and advice. If you became very ill, you could call a physician or healer—a man or a woman, university-educated or empirically trained—to look at your urine, feel your pulse, and prescribe medicines. If you had retained menses (i.e., your period was late), you might ask the nuns for an herbal tea that would start the bleeding. If you needed a finger amputated or blood letting, you might go to the barber-surgeon. (In many places, barbers were the go-to professionals for anything that involved minor cutting. They already had the razors and knew how to use them.) If you caught syphilis and were poor, you might have to go to a pox hospital, where you would be cared for by live-in nurses—usually men if you were a man, women if you were a woman. If you were having a baby, you'd send for the midwife, who would know the best labor positions to ease pain and how to slap a blue baby pink. If you were very well-off, perhaps you'd find a wet-nurse, who would not only nurse your baby with her own milk, but would also tend to its health. If your elderly husband became bedridden, and you had the means, you might hire a home nurse who could bathe and feed him. Both men and women provided health care of all kinds, and they did so in both domestic and public settings, though women practitioners were more common, and indispensable, in at-home care.

Up until the mid-Middle Ages, health care was a largely unregulated marketplace, as it had been since antiquity, one in which reputation and word-of-mouth meant a lot and in which skills could be gained through family or apprenticeship—learning by doing. Health care was very commonly provided by women, but the care was not necessarily nursing just because a woman was providing it. Strict delineation of types of care (medical, nursing, pharmaceutical) is a hallmark of our current system, but those distinctions didn't exist in the same way in the past. It was not always possible to say a given practitioner practiced *only* medicine or *only* nursing, because these artificial dividing lines had yet to be drawn.

Here is an inflection point: The first university medical schools were founded, and—with the notable exception of the University of Salerno—women weren't allowed in. Men who didn't have the necessary money or opportunity couldn't attend, either. What followed was a slow-motion cleaving of the old world of passed-down, empirical expertise from a new world of stricter hierarchy, with diplomas and licenses and legal delineations of scope. Gradually, across Europe, it became illegal to provide health care without a medical school license. Many people—but women in particular—didn't even have that option. This meant that a great swath of health care providers was practicing illegally or, at best, in a legal gray area.

If unlicensed people wanted to practice, they'd have to risk the consequences, which many did, or find an officially sanctioned way. For women, with some exceptions, those official choices evolved into nursing as a nun; practicing as a midwife, at least until the development of obstetrics; or doing the most difficult, hands-on bodywork in hospitals—anything except being the authority.

The shift was in the privileging of a certain kind of knowledge—the kind that elite men found in books, theories that were inaccessible to most—and in the suppressing of the knowledge of oral traditions; of formulas jotted down and passed on; of procedures learned by sense, by hand, by apprenticeship. This shift didn't happen all at once; it was slow but relentless. It meant the utter devaluing and even criminalization of much long-cultivated knowledge, including skilled health care practiced by women. And that is how the medical hierarchy eventually became codified: Male physicians to the top; everyone else, and women by definition, to the bottom. Historians Vern and Bonnie Bullough, PhDs, RNs, summarize the inflection point like this: "What began to separate the healer and nurse from the physician was the exclusion of women from the universities."

Women continued to practice nursing and medicine at home and in their communities; often, they could get away with it if what they were doing seemed domestic, such as midwifery or charity work. Historian Monica H. Green, PhD, has studied this shift extensively. She wrote that, in fourteenth-century Valencia, women were forbidden from providing medical care upon penalty of being whipped, but that a statute left a loophole: "They may care for little children, and women, to whom however they may give no potion." Delineations among *types* of care suddenly became central to the hierarchy. This was the seed of the modern idea that female nurses work under male physicians, who are seen as the ones with the knowledge and power. Nevertheless, women's expertise could not be erased.

Many of these medieval women practitioners had something the physicians didn't necessarily have: the trust of their communities. The early university-educated physicians were often interlopers in an established system. They had book learning, and they had status, but they didn't actually have more or different medicines, practices, or proofs than the nuns or the barbers or the lady who attended all the births. Everyone was still practicing with the theory of the humors; it wasn't as though medieval physicians had an MRI machine or chemotherapy or antibiotics. Also, physicians were expensive, there were not very many of them at first, and people did not just naturally abandon the ways they had always done things to flock, en masse, to these pricey new practitioners.

Because of this, physicians had to wage an all-out, centuries-long campaign to invent a difference between them and other health care practitioners. From the beginning, they cloaked their quest to eliminate the competition in concern over patient safety. Historian Sara Ritchey, PhD, has examined the ways that women practitioners were disappeared or neutralized. "One way that physicians sought to distinguish their practices from those of women," she writes, "was by caricaturing women healers as chatty, gullible hacks who spout futile words and wield spurious herbs." The reality was that women were no more likely to be incompetent quacks than anyone else. The story of Jacoba Felicie, a popular health care provider in fourteenth-century Paris, sheds light on how little patient safety had to do with any of it.

In 1322, the faculty of the Paris School of Medicine brought Felicie to court and accused her of practicing unofficially, which she was because she was a woman. In her own defense, she asked the court to consider the spirit of the law. She did not quibble with the medical men's desire to rid the city of quacks. In fact, in a surviving translation of the court case, she agreed that "ignorant women and inexperienced fools, untrained in the medical art," should not be allowed to practice. But this did not apply to her, she argued, because she was "expert in the art of medicine."

She brought eight witnesses to court, each one testifying to her abilities. Witness Jean Faber told the court how Felicie had success-fully treated him: "He was suffering from a certain sickness in his head and ears at a time of great heat . . . Jacoba had visited him and shown great care for him that he was cured from his illness by the potations which she gave him." A friar of the hospital in Paris testified that "he had been seized by a severe illness, to such an extent that his own limbs could not support him. . . . He had had himself taken to the house of said Jacoba . . . He was completely restored to health." He said she gave him medicinal herbs like chamomile leaves and melilot.

A woman named Jeanne said that Felicie saved her life after physicians said there was nothing they could do for her. "She had been seized by a fever, and very many physicians had visited her . . . And she was so weighed down by the said illness that on a certain Tuesday . . . she was not able to speak, and the said physicians gave her up for dead. And so it would have been, if the said Jacoba had not come to her at her request. When she had come, she inspected her urine and felt her pulse and afterwards gave her a certain clear liquid to drink, and gave her also a syrup, so that she would go to the toilet. And Jacoba so labored over her that by the grace of God she was cured of the said illness."

None of these tributes to patient safety mattered: Felicie was guilty by definition. She had charged for her services, and she had doled out medicines, acts that put her firmly in a medical professional category. She was a threat precisely because her practice was so sim-ilar to that of the official physicians. She was fined sixty livres and excommunicated, one of six unofficial medical providers (three other women and two men) to be fined and excommunicated that month.

Excommunication was an incredibly harsh sentence. The Church was at the center of European medieval life: laws were made by the Church, the government ran in concert with the Church, the community's social life was arranged around the Church. To be excommunicated was to be shunned. Some thought it worse than execution, because it ended your eternal life.

In court, Felicie described herself as an expert in medicine, not nursing, though there were elements of nursing in her practice. Whatever they called themselves, women like her were now out of a job—or, at least, one they could practice in the open. Still, physicians didn't have the desire or the ability to provide *all* the health care necessary—there weren't enough of them, and they charged fees many people could not afford. And elite physicians were not going to spend all day at the pox hospital, draining sores.

And, perhaps, this is what happened: It's not that nursing is naturally done by women, and it's not that nursing didn't exist before physicians and hospitals. It's that the new health care *structure* presented a predicament: physicians wanted to be in charge but could not provide all the health care, and there was an enduring pool of skilled workers in female practitioners. And, so, a concept of a different kind of care, an essentially female, subordinate care, started to develop. It's not that these ideas had never existed before, but this was when they became codified, even by law, into what would become today's health care hierarchy.

Such laws ushered in a dangerous time to be a female practitioner, as Felicie discovered. Even being a nun was not always a guarantee of safety for those who nursed. Nursing nuns' religious status gave them some cover, but they also had to contend with Church politics, and some walked a dangerous line regarding how much healing power and independence they could claim for themselves.

Sister Orsola, of a Benedictine convent in Pistoia, Italy, was known for visions and mystic healing powers, a charismatic mix of medicine with religious magic. Everyone who was anyone wanted Sister Orsola's remedies and her advice. To an uncomfortably pregnant archduchess, she sent medicinal spices and some blessed bread in an amulet, a talisman to soothe discomfort. She rose to become the abbess of the convent.

When the Italian Plague spread across northern Italy in the summer of 1630, Abbess Orsola started giving away water from the convent's well that she said had been blessed by Saint Benedict; she claimed the potion would prevent the plague. Crowds gathered, attracting too much attention to Orsola. The Holy Office opened an inquest. Orsola was found guilty of simulating sanctity—that is, faking the magic. She had claimed too much power for a nun. But the Church's objection wasn't to the idea that well water could miraculously prevent plague; its objection was that the miracle was Orsola's. Her writings were burned, and she was imprisoned until she died, nine years later.

She was not the only one. This kind of persecution was part of a centuries-long campaign, starting in the 1300s, in which female health care workers were maligned and scapegoated in Europe and in the European colonies. The spectrum of vilification ranged from accusations of idiot quackery to arrests for simulating holiness or practicing witchcraft to serve the Devil. Some women were especially targeted—in particular, witch-hunters spun elaborate and macabre fantasies about midwives. These efforts to link female health care workers to witchcraft make it clear that anxiety over female healing authority was high.

The *Malleus Maleficarum* (translated as *Hammer of Witches*), published under a decree by Pope Innocent VIII in 1486, was written by two prominent clergymen who were also inquisitors. It is a handbook for witch-hunting, full of lurid fantasies about the ways that women were extra-susceptible to the Devil because of their uncontrollable lust. Witches were thought to have extra nipples to suckle demons, or to be able to milk a knife or make a man's penis disappear. Demonologists argued that midwives were particularly suspect because they could harvest babies for the Devil. The *Malleus*

Maleficarum devotes an entire chapter to the many gruesome ways midwives might eat or sacrifice infants: "That in Various Ways Midwife Sorceresses Kill the Fetuses in the Womb and Cause Miscarriages, And When They Do Not Do This, They Offer the Newborns to Demons." (This is similar to the anti-Semitic tropes that were also used to target Jewish people.) It is not clear that midwives were actually disproportionately arrested for witchcraft in comparison to other women—but it is clear that their very authority was painted as a threat. Even midwives' routine practices put them at risk: inquisitors wondered if they used black magic to ease the pain of childbirth. It didn't help that midwives provided women with birth control, abortion, and family planning, an endeavor that has always put women on the wrong side of powerful men. And it was certainly true that every childbirth was (and is) rife with opportunity for things to go very wrong, with no explanation—a devilish capriciousness. "Even an innocent midwife whose patient had an unwanted result, such as a stillborn or malformed infant, was at risk of being accused of witchcraft," writes medical historian William Minkowski, MD.

Some groups of midwives were more likely to be targeted than others. Scotland saw a disproportionately high number of people accused of witchcraft. In 1590, Scottish midwife Agnes Sampson was accused of being a witch by a servant girl, who was herself accused. King James I was obsessed with witch-hunting, and he personally participated in Sampson's torture. She confessed to using magic to take away the pain of women in childbirth and said that witches sailed in sieves to meet with the Devil and plot the downfall of the king. Sampson, like other executed Scottish women, was strangled to death before being burned.

This suppression moved along predictable, overlapping lines of gender, race, and colonialism. It makes a terrible kind of sense that an instance when traditional midwives *were* brutally and disproportionately arrested by inquisitors en masse was in the Spanish colonization of "New Spain," in what is now Mexico, parts of the United States, much of Central America, and parts of northern South America. Colonizing missionaries worked with the Inquisition, importing European demonology, with which they condemned native midwives, nurses, and healers, part of an effort to suppress all indigenous culture.

Paula de Eguiluz was the rare healer who managed to use her skills and sheer nerve to subvert the process meant to destroy her. Born in 1592 in what is now the Dominican Republic to an enslaved mother and a free father, both of African descent, de Eguiluz became free in her thirties and began working as a healer, a practitioner of Afro-Caribbean love magic, and an interpreter of dreams and visions. Her healing services were popular and drew attention. Her neighbors accused her of murdering a baby by sucking on its belly button and making a pact with the Devil. She was hauled before the Inquisition in Cartagena, Colombia, where she at first denied the charges of witchcraft but later confessed. (She said a demon appeared to her as a "well-spoken white man.") She was sentenced to two hundred lashes and an auto-da-fé, a public ritual of humiliation—but she was also condemned to work for free for a time in the hospital in Cartagena, providing nursing care, tacit acknowledgment of her skill.

Even after her conviction, de Eguiluz refused to stop practicing her charismatic healing, and her services were so in demand that she became wealthy and traveled around Cartagena carried in a litter while dressed in beautiful golden clothing. She was repeatedly arrested and charged with witchcraft, but she learned how to confess and repent effectively, weaving lurid tales that out-demonologied the demonologists. And though the inquisitors continued to imprison, whip, and condemn her, they also, incredibly, sought out her treatments. With the cooperation of the inquisitors, she stayed at the home of one ill man for more than twenty days, nursing him herself while decked in a veil decorated with coral, instead of the penitential habit she was supposed to wear. Her treatments were so popular that at one auto-da-fé, the cheers and jeers of a supportive crowd drowned out the voices of the inquisitors as they intoned her crimes.

De Eguiluz was not alone in her work: her practice existed within a long Afro-Caribbean healing tradition that was suppressed by inquisitors, who called it devilish. In the *Journal of Advanced Nursing*, Diana-Lyn Baptiste, DNP, RN, and several coauthors write about how de Eguiluz fits into the larger story of nursing, a part that colonizers tried to eradicate: "De Eguiluz represents the struggles of many undocumented BIPOC nurses who were healers, doctresses and health practitioners building the foundation for nursing practice that was deemed unacceptable during this era."

In the end, the demonologists—working alongside the larger physicians' movement to suppress women's healing authority—did succeed in linking the concept of the midwife, the wisewoman, the herbalist, the nurse, and the folk medicine practitioner with witchcraft and dangerous quackery. It's one of the false stereotypes of a nurse as a witchy battle-axe, a superstitious purveyor of "old wives' tales," a joke, or a monster. In ways both subtle and very much not, that stereotype has served to discredit both nurses' and women's knowledge.

When physicians cracked down on women's healing authority, it had a devastating effect on the idea of nursing itself. Despite the long, sophisticated history of nursing, what followed the Middle Ages was an actual and/or perceived decline in the quality of nursing care that continued into the early modern period; nurses were denied education, and the hierarchy dictated that nursing was mostly a low-status endeavor. By 1844, when Dickens wrote in *Martin Chuzzlewit* of the archetypal nurse Sarah "Sairey" Gamp, a lazy, stupid old lady who reeks of rum and doesn't care if her patients live or die, her character was already a popular and familiar stereotype. Contrast it, for example, with the ancient Indian conception of a nurse as an incredibly capable person with a sterling character; or with the trained Byzantine nurses without whom the Pantokrator could not have run. History had been rewritten. It served the victors.

"The physician had become all powerful and dominant—so powerful that historians could simply overlook medieval nursing," nurse historians Vern and Bonnie Bullough write. "When educated women did enter the field again, as women nurses did in the nineteenth century, they were able to do so because they emphasized that women were 'natural' caregivers and healers." The new story—that it is natural for physicians to always be in charge and natural for women to assist them by nursing—is entirely contradicted by the actual history of nursing. And maybe that's one reason that history has been so elided.

It's easy to imagine this dynamic as a relic of the past. Women are certainly no longer barred from practicing health care—the majority of medical students are now women—or burned at the stake. But what is shockingly durable is the idea that nurses are unreliable and not well educated and therefore must be mediated and surveilled by physicians.

When the American Medical Association, a professional group for physicians, was founded in 1847, it immediately busied itself with casting midwives and other "irregular" medical providers as hacks and abortionists—shades of selling babies to the Devil. The group most especially targeted Black and immigrant midwives. And again, this was as much about competition as anything else: obstetrics was a new specialty, and midwives were taking most of the business.

This territorialism continues today. Witness, for instance, a now-deleted tweet from the American Medical Association from late 2020.

The tweet showed Scrabble tiles spelling out "NP" (nurse practitioner), "CRNA" (certified registered nurse anesthetist), and "PA" (physician assistant). Superimposed on the image are the words "Stop scope creep…because patient safety isn't a game." *Scope creep* is the sinister-sounding term the AMA uses to describe instances in which other specially trained clinicians provide care that is usually associated with physicians—such as advanced practice nurses working to the full extent of their licenses: delivering babies and caring for children, providing anesthesia, diagnosing illnesses and prescribing medications, managing chronic conditions, providing vaccines, prescribing birth control, performing physicals, and offering preventative care.

The AMA tweet inspired an immediate backlash and was taken down, but it reflects the attitude of the physicians' professional group, which has actively lobbied against efforts at the state and federal level to allow advanced practice nurses to work without physician "supervision." In twenty-four states, physicians must sign off on much of what nurse practitioners do, meaning the nurses have restricted or reduced practice authority. In many cases, this means the nurses must pay physicians thousands of dollars for collaborative practice agreements that allow them to work. Sometimes, these collaborating physicians are not even on site. In 2022, Kansas became the twenty-sixth state to lift the requirement for nurse practitioners to have physician oversight, giving nurse practitioners full-practice authority—meaning they can see patients independently, run tests and diagnose, and prescribe medicines, working to the full scope of their licenses. The patchwork of state laws is particularly nonsensical, because nurse practitioners in full-practice states like Kansas, Massachusetts, and Wyoming have the same education and training as those in restricted-practice states like Michigan, Texas, and Florida. Nevertheless, the AMA says allowing advanced practice nurses full scope of practice will result in "reduced safety for patients."

Many individual physicians have a more nuanced view of this than does their professional organization. None of this means that nurses are inherently good and physicians are inherently bad, but it does show that there are overarching power dynamics in our health care system that do not serve the patient. No one is saying someone who is not specifically qualified should be removing your gallbladder. But the AMA's insistence that physicians alone should dominate every kind of care, even when other providers are also trained and licensed to perform the same procedures, only limits the amount of care available. Also, it is not based in all the evidence—studies have shown that nurses are not just safe health care providers, but excellent ones.

Randomized clinical trials have shown that people who received their primary care from a nurse practitioner had the *same* outcomes as people who received their primary care from a physician. In fact, the U.S. Department of Veterans Affairs gave nurse practitioners full-practice authority in 2017; the department subsequently ran a study of 806,434 patients and found that primary care provided by MDs and NPs did not differ in quality, cost, or outcome. Another VA study found that there *was* a difference: "Although NPs were perceived as comparable to physicians in many ways, we found a distinct difference in patients' satisfaction and preference for the holistic, interpersonal care provided by NPs." In other words, patients often *prefer* nurse practitioner care because of the distinct ways that nurses practice. Even the National Academy of Medicine has called for ending physician oversight of advanced practice nurses in order to meet the needs of the public.

That's because fewer and fewer Americans have a primary care provider at all, and people who don't get primary care live shorter, sicker lives. In many rural areas, there is a shortage of primary care providers. In this context, why would the AMA want to further limit the number of people who can provide this much-needed care?

Writing in *The Journal for Nurse Practitioners*, Marilyn Edmunds, PhD, NP, proposed a reason. "The American Medical Association . . . has often been negative about NPs, painting all of us with the same broad brush as dangerous dabblers or incompetents who require direct supervision to protect patients. . . . To be honest, most of the AMA fight has been designed to keep NPs tied to physician practices so reimbursement for NP services goes through physicians." In short, she argues that money in health care flows through physicians, and the physicians' professional group would like to keep it that way. The group may truly believe that nurse-led care is dangerous, but the fact is that pushing that belief serves them in more ways than one. Same as it ever was.

Dangerous dabblers and incompetents. There is a direct line from the AMA's lobbying against nurse practitioners back to the faculty of the Paris School of Medicine that persecuted Jacoba Felicie based on her identity, not the evidence. And yet, none of this was inevitable, and it doesn't have to be this way. But to move forward into a future in which everyone can get the care they need, we will need to understand nursing differently.

The following chapters will bring us backward and forward in time, highlighting nurses who created or are creating that better world through their nursing, in acts of reimagination.

CHAPTER 3

IDENTITY

Who Is a Nurse? The Wartime Struggle for the Right to Care

...From the stump of the arm, the amputated hand,
I undo the clotted lint, remove the slough, wash off
*   the matter and blood,*
Back on his pillow the soldier bends with curv'd
*   neck and side falling head,*
His eyes are closed, his face is pale, he dares not look
*   on the bloody stump,*
And has not yet look'd on it....
... I am faithful, I do not give out,
The fractur'd thigh, the knee, the wound in the
*   abdomen,*
These and more I dress with impassive hand, (yet
*   deep in my breast a fire, a burning flame.)*

—"THE WOUND-DRESSER,"
WALT WHITMAN, CIVIL WAR NURSE

In early 1945, Major General Paul Hawley told the *New York Times* that eleven hospital units were arriving in the European war zone without a single nurse. Army field hospitals that already had nurses were woefully understaffed. "How much nursing care do you think that 74 nurses can give to 3,000 patients?" Hawley asked. It was a national emergency, a PR disaster. Under pressure, President Roosevelt sought solutions. Parents of soldiers fighting the Nazis feared there wouldn't be anyone to save their sons' lives if they were injured.

Newly graduated from nursing school, Nancy Leftenant-Colon, RN, went eagerly to the recruiting office. She remembers seeing a poster there, with the image of a blonde nurse standing heroically tall, wearing a white dress and cap with a blue cape around her shoulders: NURSES ARE NEEDED NOW!

This moment was the culmination of Leftenant-Colon's childhood dreams. All her life, she had had two goals. "I always wanted to be a nurse," she said, sitting in the library at Dominican Village, a retirement and assisted living community in Amityville, New York, aged one hundred, wearing crisp jeans and a blouse, her silver hair in a flawless bouffant. "And I wanted to go into the service. I always had the military on my mind. That was my goal, and I wouldn't settle for anything less than that."

Leftenant-Colon was born in Amityville, where she grew up one of twelve children in a tight-knit, religious family. After graduating from high school, she wanted to attend Lincoln School for Nurses in the Bronx, the most well-regarded nursing school for Black women at the time. To save money for the tuition, she worked for ten dollars a week at her local hospital, scrubbing floors and washing dishes. She would walk the two miles home at night when she missed the last bus. She can't remember exactly how long it took her to save enough for nursing school, but it was a very long time. Finally, when she had enough, she enrolled. She graduated from Lincoln in the midst of

World War II, as news of the dire nurse shortage in the armed forces was making headlines across the country. But when she presented herself at the recruiting office, they said they weren't taking nurses. They said to forget it, to go home. Leftenant-Colon knew that what they meant was that they weren't taking *Black* nurses. But she was not going to take no for an answer.

When a country is at war, its fortunes often rise and fall on the fitness of its troops—in other words, wars can be won or lost on nursing. When governments restrict who can nurse for their countries, they essentially withhold full citizenship from those nurses. (And in doing so, they hurt their own war effort.) And so, the fight to nurse during war is the fight for equal rights. Leftenant-Colon knew herself to be an American and a nurse. Her country's refusal to let her serve indicated that her country did not consider her a real American or a real nurse. At the time, nursing existed within a segregated country with a segregated armed forces and a segregated health care system. But on top of that, nursing leadership, in a drive to define professional modern nursing, had itself leveraged racial, gender, and class bias to distinguish this new profession from what had been done for millennia by all kinds of skilled people—men and women of all races—from around the world.

Leftenant-Colon would eventually become one of the first Black nurses to serve in the U.S. Army Nurse Corps and the first to serve as a regular member when the military officially desegregated. How she got there is a collective story of struggle and determination, a story that has one origin all the way back in the Crimean War in 1854, when Florence Nightingale and her contemporaries tried to enforce an idea that some people were nurses and some people were not.

The leaders who codified modern nursing in the 1800s believed that not everyone *could* be a real nurse. To them, being a nurse was not just about skills and education; it was about moral purity. And this weaponized status was available only to certain women—white, Christian, mostly middle- or upper-class. And so, though they carved out a role for *some* women in modern health care, leaders like Florence Nightingale in England and Dorothea Dix in the United States also explicitly shut out others. "Those that started this nascent profession, started nursing schools, believed that the only people who could attain that high standard of morality was a very specific group of women, and that was often defined by race and class," said historian Charissa J. Threat, PhD, author of *Nursing Civil Rights*, a definitive book on the intersection of gender and race in military nursing. Men were entirely left out, despite their long history of providing care. When nurse pioneers argued that caring was an immutably feminine characteristic, they also went right along with the very essentialist ideas that kept women subjugated.

Nightingale is probably the most famous nurse who ever lived, but she had a less-celebrated contemporary: Mary Seacole. The two women's motivations for wanting to serve in the Crimean War of 1853-56 were parallel, but the legacies of their wartime nursing are remarkably different. Those differences are telling, even today. Both Nightingale and Seacole were experienced nurses, though with vastly different styles and goals. Both were deeply moved by patriotism and compassion to nurse British soldiers during the notoriously bloody war fought mainly on the Crimean Peninsula, in what is now Russian-occupied Ukraine. One became heralded as the founder of modern nursing; the other was mostly forgotten—or condescendingly referred to as "the Black Nightingale," her story asterisked in relation to others'. In *The Satanic Verses*, Salman Rushdie remarks upon this contrast: "Here is Mary Seacole, who did as much in the Crimea as another magic-lamping lady, but, being dark, could scarce be seen for the flame of Florence's candle."

Seacole was born in 1805 in Kingston, Jamaica, under colonial

British rule. Her father was a long-gone Scottish solider, and her mother was a well-known Afro-Caribbean "doctress" who ran a boarding house/clinic in the capital. Seacole grew up watching her mother treat both locals and British officers and practiced the remedies on her dolls. She always had extraordinary wanderlust. (Her autobiography is aptly and marvelously titled *Wonderful Adventures of Mrs Seacole in Many Lands*.) As a young woman, she sailed with relatives to visit London and then, later, to the Bahamas, Cuba, and Haiti. Back in Kingston, she married a Mr. Seacole—"Poor man! He was very delicate"—who quickly sickened and died despite her nursing. She never remarried, though she was at pains to make it clear that her singleness was by choice. After her mother died, Seacole built her own fortune in Kingston as a healer: "I had gained a reputation as a skillful nurse and doctoress, and my house was always full of invalid officers and their wives."

When a cholera epidemic swept through Jamaica in 1850, Seacole became adept at treating the disease, using techniques she had learned from a Dr. B., who was lodging with her. Later, she was visiting her brother in Cruces, Panama, when cholera came again. Seacole described her work during this outbreak in a passage that makes clear the pride she took in her skill: "Selecting from my medicine chest—I never travel anywhere without it—what I deemed necessary, I went hastily to the patient and at once adopted the remedies I considered fit. It was a very obstinate case, but by dint of mustard emetics, warm fomentations, mustard plasters on the stomach and the back and calomel, at first in large and then in gradually smaller doses, I succeeded in saving my first cholera patient in Cruces."

When the Crimean War broke out, Seacole was consumed with the news of it; she had many friends in the British Army, as these soldiers were her regular patients in Jamaica. The war had started between the Turkish Ottoman Empire and the Russians in 1853, and by 1854, the British and French had been drawn into it, fighting with the Turks against the Russians. The conflict was ostensibly about the rights of Christian minorities in the Ottoman Empire, but it was really about Russian expansionism and the power vacuum that the decline of the Ottoman Empire would leave in Europe and Central Asia. The fighting centered on the then-Russian-held Crimean Peninsula, a long-contested part of the world, valuable for its fertile soil and large Black Sea port city, Sevastopol, which has access to the Mediterranean Sea through the Bosphorus Strait.

Officials promised, as they often do, that the war would be over soon, in just a matter of weeks, but the war dragged on, with horrific numbers of casualties. Word reached Britain of needless deaths, soldiers dying with no one to care for them. Infectious diseases ripped through the army; every wound suppurated. The British military hospitals in Scutari, Turkey (present-day Uskudar), near the fighting, were full, there were not enough physicians or orderlies, and conditions were so squalid as to be dangerous. "The brave fellows," Seacole wrote, "were dying thousands of miles away from the active sympathy of their fellow countrymen."

This crisis was what finally led the British War Office to contract with female nurses for the first time, under Nightingale's leadership. Seacole wanted to join up. "What delight should I not experience if I could be useful to my own 'sons,' suffering for a cause it was so glorious to fight and bleed for!" she writes, referring, as she often did, to the British soldiers as her sons and to herself as their mother. "I made up my mind that if the army wanted nurses, they would be glad of me." This was a completely logical conclusion: Soldiers in Crimea were dying as much of illness as of war injury, struck with cholera, diarrhea, and dysentery, all of which Seacole had been treating her whole life. In fact, she had already once been hired by the British Army in Jamaica to organize nurses in response to a yellow fever epidemic on the island.

So Seacole showed up at the London War Office to volunteer as a Crimean hospital nurse. The secretary at war, Sidney Herbert, would not see her, so she went to the quartermaster-general's office, where a man suggested she apply to the medical department. But when she showed up there, they would not see her, either. So, she decided to go straight to Nightingale and offer herself as a recruit. To do this, she needed to see Elizabeth Herbert, the wife of the very secretary at war who had already rejected her.

Herbert was handling Nightingale's ongoing recruiting out of her own home, so Seacole got the address and "laid pernicious siege" to the house. She came prepared with references—like one from a British medical officer from a gold-mining company in Grenada, testifying to her nursing skills. She sat for a very long time, pointedly ignored. She noticed that people in the house seemed to resent her presence: "[They] marveled exceedingly at the yellow woman whom no excuses could get rid of, nor impertinence dismay." Imagine her: Seacole had a broad, expressive face with a lined forehead and deep-set eyes. She dressed well, with lace collars and earrings and ample corseted dresses on her stout form, curly dark hair severely parted down the middle and pulled back. As she was, she sat, and waited.

Finally, "Mrs. H" sent a message: Actually, they were not hiring any more nurses. Seacole knew what this meant. Still, she went back on a subsequent day, when she was told the same thing: They didn't need any nurses. "And I read in her face the fact that, had there been a vacancy, I should not have been chosen to fill it," Seacole writes. The army did need nurses, and Nightingale was still recruiting, but they didn't want *her*.

Seacole wrote of the grief of this moment: "I was . . . so certain of the service I could render among the sick soldiery, and yet I found it so difficult to convince others of those facts . . . Was it possible that American prejudices against colour had some root here? Did these ladies shrink from accepting my aid because my blood flowed beneath a somewhat duskier skin than theirs? Tears streamed down my foolish cheeks, as I stood in the fast-thinning streets; tears of grief that any should doubt my motives."

Seacole's generous assumption that her expertise would be welcome must have been based in experience. She had been traveling and working in racially mixed communities her whole life, and in her book, she notes when she experienced racism—such as when a group of Americans in Panama did not want to share a boat with her. But it was painful for her to ascribe the same bias to British people; she was patriotic and, in many ways, considered *herself* British.

Nightingale *certainly* considered herself British, and—in contrast to Seacole—so did everyone else. Nightingale was a well-connected Londoner, a wealthy, highly educated political insider who ran in circles of government officials and their wives. She had trained in nursing at the Deaconess Institute of Kaiserswerth, Germany, a Lutheran nursing school founded in 1836. Then, unmarried in her thirties, she supervised a small London hospital for women. She did this for free—a woman of her class did not take a paying job.

Nightingale became Nightingale when, in the fall of 1854, the crisis of care in Crimea became sensational news. The *Times* war correspondent in Constantinople wrote that the British soldiers in the war hospitals had no nurses, no bandages, and were "left to expire in agony." This was the first war with regular photojournalism and correspondence, and the resulting transparency was deeply upsetting for the public. The very next day, the same *Times* correspondent asked why the British did not have their own nursing service, as the French did in the Sisters of Charity. The British government was suddenly very much on the spot. The secretary *at* war, Sidney Herbert, immediately thought of Florence Nightingale. He suggested to the

Duke of Newcastle, Henry Pelham-Clinton, the secretary of state *for* war, that perhaps Britain *did* need something like the French had—and perhaps Florence Nightingale could lead it.

Newcastle liked the idea. Both he and Herbert knew Nightingale and her family. But despite being totally overwhelmed, British military physicians did not want female nurses, whom they thought of as drunk and callous—like Dickens's Sairey Gamp. They weren't particularly mollified by Nightingale's social class because they found the idea of a lady mixing in the outside work of men appalling, especially in a war zone. But the ministers were convinced that, with her abilities and her sterling bearing and upbringing, if anyone could wrangle a socially acceptable nursing plan into action, it was Nightingale.

Meanwhile—just like Seacole—Nightingale had read about the horrors of this war and, on her own, had become galvanized to help however she could. She hatched a plan to travel to the war zone with a private group of just three or four nurses, thinking that the military physicians would be more likely to cooperate with a small, unofficial nurse cadre than a large, conspicuous one. She didn't want to be seen as overstepping. She wrote to Elizabeth Herbert, asking what she thought of this modest plan. As it happened, Sidney Herbert had just written his own letter to Nightingale, asking if she would lead an official government contingent of nurses to the military hospitals close to the war zone, in Scutari. The story goes that their letters crossed in the mail. Ultimately, Nightingale agreed to Herbert's bigger, more public plan.

Nightingale hired thirty-eight nurses for the initial group—the group Seacole wanted to join—placing special emphasis on their experience and "respectability," a tricky combination; most experienced hospital nurses were working class, and the working class was considered less respectable in Nightingale's world by definition. (More than one hundred nurses, all white women, would eventually be sent from Britain to work under Nightingale as the war ground on.)

Nightingale deployed the nurses differently based on their class. The working-class women were what she called assistant nurses; they would now be called regular bedside nurses. These nurses did much of the direct patient care, but Nightingale also put them to work in the laundry, cleaning and cooking, and she sometimes referred to them as servants. The middle-class nurses were head nurses—Nightingale felt that she could better trust them to behave respectably and enforce rules, even if they were less experienced in nursing. She also hired nuns; they were some of the most experienced (and respectable) nurses around; plus, the government wanted the nursing force to include both Catholics and Protestants, as a gesture of unity. Everyone had to agree not to proselytize. From the beginning, there was deep political meaning placed on the identities of the Nightingale nurses; the ministers were anxious that they be of unimpeachable character.

Once in Turkey, near the fighting in Crimea, Nightingale took over daily operations at the several British base hospitals in Scutari, on the Asian side of Constantinople. She would also oversee nursing care at British hospitals near Balaclava, closer to the front. (The British government also ran several other wartime hospitals where Nightingale did not direct the nursing care.) She later referred to the conditions she found in Scutari as "hell on earth." Soldiers were shipped in from the front via the Black Sea. Many were already in bad shape when they arrived, and hospital conditions were miserable: overflowing buckets of human waste, filthy bedding and bandages, blocked drainage pipes, and underneath, giant undrained sewers and unburied dead animals. The bodies of wounded men crawled with lice; infections, gangrene, and pests of all kinds were rampant. Germ theory was not yet widely understood or accepted—Nightingale was operating with miasma theory, which held that disease was spread by dirty air and bad odors. The theory wasn't right, but it held a kernel of truth: the state of the hospital was a massive health problem. She organized her nurses to clean the linens, open the windows, scrub the floors and walls, change bandages and bedding as often as possible, and clean the drains.

At first, it wasn't enough, and the death rate continued to climb. A few months later, the British government sent a sanitary commission to drain the sewers under the hospitals and remove the dead animals polluting the water supply. After that, mortality went from about 40 percent of all patients to about 2 percent. One of Nightingale's most enduring public health accomplishments was her original use of statistics to show how these sanitary measures resulted in fewer infections and deaths. (Her writings on the importance of ventilation were relevant during the Covid-19 pandemic.)

Nightingale knew that she had been hired to lead a political experiment and that some of the British Army physicians would have been happy to see her fail. Some officers found her disturbingly unladylike: for instance, she attended surgeries on naked men. The mere presence of her and her group of nurses was considered a subversion of the order of things in multiple ways: Ladies should not be hired nurses, much less in a male-dominated war zone. Ladies shouldn't mix with working-class women, who made up the majority of the hospital nurses and who were thought to be morally suspect. The nun nurses were also loath to be associated with working-class nurses; the nuns had their own, long-established nursing systems and were generally not happy to be directed by Nightingale. Nightingale was navigating Victorian anxieties around propriety, hierarchy, and women's work outside the home, all on behalf of the British government and in a war zone.

Nightingale was consumed with the desire to succeed, and she responded to the delicacy of her political situation with absolute deference to the British social order. She wanted, badly, to prove that *some* women—certain trained, sober, proper, white Christian women—could be a new kind of nurse, essential to the health of the nation. She believed that the British Empire had a god-given duty to improve the world by bringing the "uncivilized" into "civilization." Writing in the online journal *Nursing Clio*, Natalie Stake-Doucet, PhD, RN, pointed out that Nightingale "was a staunch supporter of British colonialism, even with the knowledge of the death and destruction left in its wake."

Nightingale meticulously re-created the social order within her nursing workforce. She envisioned nursing as distinct from medicine, with a female-only chain of command, but she still maintained that nurses were in service to physicians, who were at the top. She, upper-class lady nurse superintendent, took orders from them. Her middle-class head nurses came next in the hierarchy, and the working-class assistant nurses were at the bottom. She could not, would not, usurp male medical authority in the hospital, and she took this stance of total obedience as far as it could go. If a physician had not ordered water for a dying man, Nightingale would not give the man water. If a patient craved a sweet or a cordial or a biscuit, and it had not been ordered by a physician, Nightingale would decline. Obedience was the priority; providing appropriate care was important, but secondary. Nightingale's nurses were not allowed to establish rapport with the patients, because of Victorian anxieties over sex. They were not allowed to read to the patients, either—Nightingale had been explicitly tasked with ensuring that no religious or political proselytizing would occur. Nurse historian Carol Helmstadter describes this oppressive dynamic in her book *Beyond Nightingale*: "Nightingale locked all the nurses—Sisters, ladies, and working class—into the nurses' quarters at 8:30 every night and slept with the key under her pillow."

Many of the nurses found Nightingale's strict insistence on obedience cruel and contrary to the point of nursing. She fired four of six nurses from St. John House, a Catholic nurse training school in London, because they had fed patients without explicit medical orders for food. As Helmstadter uncovered, one of these nurses wrote to her superior in London, shocked by Nightingale's dictatorial style: "We do not look for many comforts, but we do feel we ought to be trusted. We are not allowed to go into the wards without one of the lady nurses. We must not speak one word of comfort to a poor dying man or read to him. We are prevented from doing what our hearts prompt us to do. We feel we are not so useful as we expected to be."

Nevertheless, when the war was over, Nightingale's experiment was considered a resounding victory—she had cleaned up the hospitals, savvily navigated the politics, and shown that sanitary nursing care and management improved outcomes. (This victory went along with the larger one: the British, French, and Ottomans had defeated the Russians.) Nightingale demonstrated to the Victorians that a select group of women could serve their country by nursing. This was, in her context, an earthquake—the idea that working outside the home was not just something that poor women did because they had no choice but that middle- and upper-class women could offer something important to the world through nursing work.

Nightingale returned home to a rapturous public and glowing press coverage. Henry Wadsworth Longfellow wrote a poem about her called "Santa Filomena," immortalizing her as "a lady with a lamp." Because of an illness, she never returned to direct-care nursing, but she raised money to start a school of nursing based on her conception of the profession. Her style of nurse training, and everything that went with it, spread around the world. Perhaps her most surprising success was that she managed to reinforce Victorian social mores while doing something that *could* have been subversive—in so doing, she crafted an ideal of nursing as a profession that was appealing to those in power. She changed the system from so far inside it that she ended up replicating it exactly.

But Nightingale was not the only woman leading a nursing corps during the Crimean War, though the others are less well remembered. The Daughters of Charity of Saint Vincent de Paul were trained Catholic nurses who provided hospital nursing for the French military, as they had done for more than two hundred years. Russia also organized a group of nurses, the Sisters of the Exaltation of the Cross, to tend casualties on the battlefield and in Crimean hospitals. The Russian sisterhood was open to women of any Christian faith and any class, and while they were at first untrained, a training program was established for them as the war went on. And Seacole was there, too.

After Seacole was turned away from Nightingale's group, she did the only thing she could do, which was to set out on her own, with the help of a business partner, for Crimea. When she arrived in Constantinople, she went to one of Nightingale's hospitals at Scutari, intending to stay only the night. But when she walked in, she saw there was work to be done and simply started doing it: "One doctor, who had with some surprise and, at first, alarm on his face, watched me replace a bandage, which was giving pain, said, very kindly when I had finished, 'Thank you, ma'am.'"

Then she went over to the nurses' quarters, where one of Nightingale's nurse managers rushed out, confused, to say that there were no job vacancies. Seacole replied that she knew that and explained that she was headed to the front the next morning; she wondered if she might spend the night. She was given a bed in the hospital's washerwomen's quarters. Ever undaunted, she enjoyed her stay: "My experience of washerwomen, all the world over, is the same—that they are kind soft-hearted folks."

From there, Seacole made her way to the outpost of Balaclava in Crimea, near the fighting, and there, she set up a shop/clinic/restaurant to aid the British soldiers. She called it the British Hotel. Sometimes her dual role as a nurse and provisioner is used to argue that she wasn't a true nurse—she was also selling chicken broth and cake and claret. But she did not have unlimited funds or a government salary. She could have sold wares and remedies anywhere, as she had in the past, but she stated that she went to Crimea to nurse, and she did—even if she was not given the official title or the respect of a nurse.

Seacole had a different nursing practice from Nightingale's. She attended to her patients in a more holistic way, one that encompassed physical, mental, and material care. We now recognize this as a key, defining feature of nursing and of patient-centered care. She saw provisioning as part of providing comfort, whether it was baking little sponge cakes for wounded men to remind them of home or bringing broth for an officer with a fever. Sometimes she even provided what we would now call palliative care, for she spent substantial time with wounded soldiers who would not survive, dabbing tea or water on their lips.

Seacole rose each day at around 4 a.m., plucked and cut up chickens for dinner, swept the floor, rolled out pastry, mixed medicines, and boiled coffee. At daybreak, men would begin to come by for coffee. Then there would be a morning rush of sick and injured people. For many hours a day, she dosed out medicines and treated broken bones, wounds, and frostbite in winter while also roasting chickens and selling boots and linens. Her British Hotel served both lunch and dinner, and the kitchen closed at 8 p.m. Seacole was careful to note this closing time, and that she did not tolerate drunkenness, cards, or dice, likely because she knew of the rumors, later spread by Nightingale, that her establishment was a place of loose morals. (After the war, in a letter to her brother-in-law, Nightingale even suggested that the British Hotel was hardly better than a brothel.)

Despite these many obstacles, Seacole was undeterred. After the Battle of the Chernaya, on August 16, 1855, she described the scene: "The ground was thickly cumbered with the wounded ... all wanting water, and grateful to those who administered it ... I attended to the wounds of many French and Sardinians and helped to lift them into the ambulances..." When the besieged city of Sevastopol fell, she was there. "I dressed the wound of one of the officers, seriously hit in the mouth; I attended to another wounded in the throat, and bandaged the hand of a third, terribly crushed by a rifle-bullet."

Like Nightingale, Seacole believed that her identity as a woman, a kind of ur-mother, was key to her ability to nurse, but she wasn't wedded to the idea that she was beneath physicians, though she certainly respected them. She wrote of her collaboration with physicians on the sick wharf of Balaclava, where the wounded waited to be evacuated: "With so many patients, the doctors must be glad of all the hands they could get. Indeed so strong was the old impulse within me, that I waited for no permission but seeing a poor artilleryman stretched upon a pallet, groaning heavily, I ran up to him at once, and eased the stiff dressings. Lightly my practiced fingers ran over the familiar work, and well was I rewarded when the poor fellow's groans subsided ... I stooped down and raised some tea to his baked lips." She waited for no permission. What could they do? Send her home? She was there in no official capacity and received no wage.

Seacole's nursing in Crimea did not receive as much notice as Nightingale's, but she did become a public figure in her own right. In 1855, the *Morning Advertiser* wrote of her wartime nursing with admiration: "Her powders for the latter [diarrhea] epidemic are now so renowned, that she is constantly beset with applications, and it must be stated, to her honor, that she makes no charges for her powders. She is often seen riding out to the front with baskets of medicines of her own preparation."

Seacole and Nightingale's roles were extremely different, and so was their scope of practice. But *why* did one go to the front with the weight of the British government behind her and the other alone and on her own dime? *Why* was one style of nursing spread all over the world and the other denigrated as mere shopkeeping? And most important, what does that mean *now*?

After the war, Seacole returned to England to find she was bankrupt as a result of having gone to Crimea. A letter to the editor of the *Times* in 1856 from a Crimean War veteran read, "While the benevolent deeds of Florence Nightingale are being handed down to posterity with blessings and imperishable renown, are the humbler actions of Mrs Seacole to be entirely forgotten, and will none now substantially testify to the worth of those services . . . ?" Eventually, British Army officers held a benefit to raise money for Seacole, and she wrote her autobiography, but she would die in relative obscurity. One group always remembered her well: in 1954, the Nurses Association of Jamaica named its headquarters the Mary Seacole House.

Seacole's story echoes. Much later, after World War II, the United Kingdom put out a call for workers from across the British colonies and the Commonwealth, particularly nurses. Caribbean nurses from the colonies answered the call and were indispensable in starting the United Kingdom's National Health Service. Many Caribbean nurses moved to the United Kingdom permanently with their families, and at the time, because they were from British colonies, there was never any question that they were legal immigrants. In 2017, however, it emerged that the government had destroyed landing cards and other documentation and had been treating some of these nurses and their children as illegal immigrants, in some cases, deporting them back to countries they had left decades earlier. These nurses had answered Britain's call, had nursed on behalf of a country they considered their home—but for some, it seemed, the status of being a British nurse was conditional.

In 2016, there was a drive to rectify Seacole's disappearance from the narrative by placing a bronze statue of her on the grounds of St Thomas' Hospital in London, the hospital where Nightingale established a school of nursing. One Nightingale scholar was so upset by the plan for the statue that she established a society with the goal of derailing the project, even though it had the backing of the Royal College of Nursing. It was a bizarre level of resistance. Nevertheless, Seacole stands at St Thomas' now, cast in bronze, striding forward, her eyes fixed on the horizon.

Nightingale, of course, was both remembered and mythologized, and her emphasis on hierarchy and propriety has permeated nursing—as seen in the often extreme rigidity of nursing education, even today, with some nursing students doing their clinical training penalized for wearing the wrong socks or having a visible tattoo or natural Black hair. Every problem can't be laid at one woman's feet, but it is important to ask what the cost has been of venerating Nightingale to the exclusion of others. She is often the only historical nurse taught about in nursing schools, perhaps leaving nurses themselves to think she's the only option to emulate. Historians have examined why Nightingale has held such singular power given that the true history of nursing is far richer and more complicated than the Nightingale lone-hero myth.

Historian Helmstadter writes that Nightingale's model quickly became dominant, but not necessarily because it was the most effective: "It was the class-structured British model, made glamorous by the socially elite Nightingale, which would become the transnational archetype after the war." The fact that Nightingale's nursing replicated the restrictive social structure is what made it so durable. Perhaps this is because nursing, in reality, is so intimate, so relationship-based, so resistant to strict categorization and hierarchy, so rooted in moments of universal vulnerability, that it is potentially subversive, especially when done by people of all backgrounds, races, and classes. Think of Seacole: making cakes, prescribing medicines learned from her Jamaican mother, *not waiting for permission*. Nightingale tamed nursing, and for some people, that was a great relief.

By the time the American Civil War began, about five years after the end of the Crimean War, Nightingale was a cross-Atlantic celebrity. Dorothea Dix, a mental health care reformer, was appointed as superintendent of army nurses, to organize nurses for Union hospitals. It was the first time the U.S. government had officially contracted with female nurses in a war effort. This was fateful—like the Crimean War, the U.S. Civil War lasted longer and was bloodier than government leaders initially hoped, and the existing system of soldier "stewards" (nurses) assigned to hospital duty would prove totally insufficient.

Even before Dix embarked on the project, the U.S. surgeon general was swamped with applicants who wanted to join up to nurse. They were nuns, grandmothers, adolescents, free Black people, farm wives, immigrants, and well-off ladies. Dix, who admired Nightingale so much that she had traveled all the way to Turkey to meet her, only to find she had already left, wasn't having it. Following what she saw as the Nightingale model, she stipulated that nurses must be women between about ages thirty and fifty and "very plain looking" and must wear black or brown dresses—no hoop skirts, no jewelry, no bows, and no curls. "Sober, earnest and self-sacrificing" were job qualifications, and applicants needed letters of reference testifying to their morality. Dix also hired only white women and wanted only those who could afford to volunteer, though the government would later offer wages to some.

Dix certainly aspired to be Nightingale's American counterpart, but there were differences between them. For one thing, Dix wasn't seeking candidates with nursing experience, so she avoided the dilemma posed by most experienced nurses' being working class. She was also anti-Catholic and wouldn't work with nuns, which eliminated the other large group of experienced nurses. As with Nightingale, many army physicians wanted Dix to fail—but unlike Nightingale, she was willing to openly spar with them. In her efforts to prove those physicians wrong, she tried to emulate Nightingale's example, believing that strict propriety above all else would bring her success, that nursing was a moral endeavor that only *certain* women could perform. She expected the nurses to be in their beds, lights out, at 9 p.m., unless they were working. She even turned down one of the only woman physicians in the country, who volunteered to nurse, because she did not meet the age requirement. Eventually, Dix hired about three thousand nurses, rejecting many who didn't meet her criteria. Louisa May Alcott made the cut, but she later wrote of Dix, "No one likes her, and I don't wonder." Clara Barton, who nursed at Civil War hospitals and battlefields and would go on to found the American Red Cross, worked independently of Dix and started nursing by simply showing up.

As Dix went about selecting nurses to her exact specifications, the Civil War escalated, with mounting bloodshed. All told, 750,000 soldiers would be killed—2.5 percent of the total American population—and more than half a million wounded. It is still the bloodiest war the United States ever fought. The number of soldiers involved was much larger than that in the Crimean War, and in this violent, sprawling context, Dix's narrow definition of nursing was rendered absurd against the enormity of the need.

After the carnage of Gettysburg, the U.S. surgeon general went around Dix and authorized all Union Army surgeons to appoint nurses for the war effort. The reality was that the nursing landscape of the Civil War was already tumultuous. People who did not meet Dix's eligibility requirements found ways to nurse anyway, often by simply doing it, as Barton did, or by leveraging other connections to get appointed. That's not to say it was simple or the same for everyone: in the South, enslaved people were *forced* to nurse.

For instance, Henry Martin, a Civil War nurse, had been born enslaved to Thomas Jefferson and was sold away from Monticello and his family to settle Jefferson's debts. As a young man, Martin was enslaved at the University of Virginia, working as a dormitory caretaker. When the war broke out, university buildings were used as Confederate hospitals, and Martin worked as a nurse. After, as a free man, he continued to work at the university for more than four decades, as the bell ringer. In a 1914 yearbook interview, he remembered nursing hundreds of wounded young men in the university's grand Rotunda. "When I go in now," he said, "I'm thinking on the soldiers that I seen laying on the floor."

In both the Union and the Confederacy, many nursed for more than one reason—the desire to care, for recognition, to be useful, or to be able to travel with a beloved solider. The need for a wage was also a factor, though some well-off women volunteered and refused the money. The tumult of the war and the newness of official army nursing sometimes made it hard for nurses to receive their salaries. Black women especially struggled to get paid at all.

The poet and journalist Walt Whitman was drawn into nursing for the Union when he saw his brother's name on a list of the injured and raced to Fredericksburg, Virginia, to see him. His brother turned out to be fine, but the first thing Whitman saw at the hospital was a wagonful of amputated limbs. He felt compelled to stay and help, and for three years he volunteered as a nurse for the Union hospitals in the area, accompanying the wounded from Virginia to the hospitals in Washington, DC, and providing comforts (special foods or tobacco, the service of writing a letter or reading aloud) to wounded and dying soldiers. He supported himself by writing pieces for the *New York Times* and other periodicals. For the *Brooklyn Daily Eagle,* he described one of the hospitals: "Imagine a long one-story wooden shed . . . well whitewashed, then cluster ten or a dozen of these together with several smaller sheds and tents, and you have the soldiers' hospital as generally adopted here. It will contain perhaps six or seven hundred men, or perhaps a thousand, and occasionally more still." The need for nurses was that vast.

Whitman wrote the poem "The Wound-Dresser" about what he witnessed. It is unflinching in its description of what weapons do to people, the cycle of bodies destroyed by machines of war, the nurses trying desperately to mend them—a terrible push-pull of human be-havior. "I dress a wound in the side, deep, deep, / But a day or two more, for see the frame all wasted and sinking, / And the yellow-blue countenance see. / I dress the perforated shoulder, the foot with the bullet-wound, / Cleanse the one with a gnawing and putrid gangrene, so sickening, so offensive," he wrote. Whitman's wartime nursing would leave him with nightmares and flashbacks for the rest of his life.

Though male soldiers could get up to thirty dollars a month for hospital duty, Whitman was not paid, perhaps because he stood so far outside the order of things. He was not a soldier, who could nurse as a "steward," and he was not a nurse, if nurses were only women. Some accounts describe him as shunned by women nurses, perhaps because he was a man in what they thought of as a woman's sphere.

Susie King Taylor also nursed despite being denied the title and the compensation that went with it. Her official job description in the Civil War was "laundress," a designation that made her ineligible for a salary or a pension. But Taylor, who had been born enslaved, did nurse throughout the war, and she wrote in her autobiography that she was too busy with nursing to do much laundry.

Taylor had been sent to live with her grandmother in Savannah when she was a child. In the city, she went to a secret school, walking there each morning with her books wrapped in paper to hide them. She excelled and continued to study covertly as war descended upon them, with whispers of the Yankees bringing an end to slavery. She escaped when the fighting came to Savannah in 1862 and made her way to Beaufort, South Carolina, where she joined the Union's brand-new First South Carolina Volunteer Infantry Regiment, a force made up mostly of Gullah men from Georgia and South Carolina, one of the first Black regiments. (It would later be known as the Thirty-Third U.S. Colored Infantry Regiment.) There, she nursed, both in the camp and at field hospitals.

She described her work: "It seems strange how our aversion to seeing suffering is overcome in war, how we are able to see the most sickening sights, such as men with their limbs blown off and mangled by the deadly shells, without a shudder; and instead of turning away, how we hurry to assist in alleviating their pain, bind up their wounds, press the cool water to their parched lips." She also taught soldiers to read and write in her off-hours.

Harriet Tubman worked in the same regiment, as a nurse, scout, and spy. Like Taylor, Tubman was not paid for her work, and she did not receive a pension until she was nearly eighty years old, after petitioning for one for years.

But by the time World War I broke out, there was no way for American nurses to serve their country without joining the newly formed Army Nurse Corps (ANC)—the war was overseas, so no one could simply show up and start doing what needed to be done. To join the ANC, you had to join the American Red Cross, which supplied the government with qualified nurses. Black nurses showed up and volunteered, and like Seacole before them, they were met with silence.

By this point, there was a more organized system of nurse education, mostly training schools run within hospitals, and though these schools and hospitals were largely segregated, there were many qualified graduate Black nurses. (In 1879, Mary Eliza Mahoney had become the first Black nurse to graduate from an American nursing school.) Black nurses received similar educations and passed the same state board licensing exams as their non-Black counterparts.

Jane Delano, of the American Red Cross, was asked repeatedly why she would not admit Black women into the pool of qualified nurses who could be called up. She vamped on the question, claiming that she *was*, in fact, enrolling Black nurses and that she'd call them *if* there was ever an opportunity for them to serve. A month before the war ended, eighteen Black nurses were called up to serve at army camps in the United States, out of about thirty-three thousand nurses who served throughout the war.

It would take world-shaking events to get white nursing leadership, and the U.S. government, to reluctantly treat Black nurses as both full nurses and full Americans. What it took was the catastrophic nurse shortage of World War II and, with it, the very real threat of a draft on white nurses. And it took the relentless, organized struggle of an extraordinary nurse, Mabel K. Staupers, RN, who, along with her colleagues, fully understood that the desegregation of the Army Nurse Corps could be a powerful blow to Jim Crow, the system of legalized racism and segregation in force at the time.

Staupers, who was born in Barbados, was the executive secretary of the National Association of Colored Graduate Nurses (NACGN), a professional organization that existed because the American Nurses Association's chapters refused to admit Black nurses. When World War II broke out, Staupers was resolute that Black nurses would not be excluded from serving. In 1940, in the lead-up to the United States' joining the war, various nursing organizations came together to plan the provision of nurses for the potential war effort, and Black nurses were there. This inclusion left Staupers optimistic. Then she had a meeting with the surgeon general of the army, James C. Magee.

Magee already had a plan for the deployment of Black nurses: he'd allow fifty-six Black nurses to serve, just enough to staff segregated hospital wards at army bases in the U.S. South, where large numbers of Black servicemen were based. In other contexts, he didn't see a reason to staff Black nurses; he believed in segregation. Historian Darlene Clark Hine, PhD, recounts how McGee defended the policy: He "would not place white soldiers in the position where they would have to accept service from Negro professionals." Meanwhile, the navy refused to allow Black nurses to serve at all. (The air force was not yet a separate branch and was included in the army.)

There were about nine thousand Black graduate nurses in the United States at the time, and many wanted to serve. When Staupers heard that only fifty-six would be allowed into the U.S. Army Nurse Corps, she knew she would have to organize. That number was barely an improvement on the handful of Black nurses who had served in World War I, but it was the tiniest opening. She gathered Black leaders around the issue, all of them cognizant of the potential symbolic and material importance of the inclusion of Black nurses in the war effort. Staupers was a masterful publicist, and she put out a steady stream of press releases calling the paltry, segregated quota to attention, and Black newspapers around the country covered the issue extensively. Hine uncovered a letter from Staupers to Mary Beard, the director of the American Red Cross Nursing Service, that reads, "We fail to understand how America can say to the world that in this country we are ready to defend democracy when its Army and Navy are committed to a policy of discrimination."

Meanwhile, the army's system of segregation badly complicated care on the ground. Prudence Burns Burrell, RN, was one of the first Black nurses to get one of the few quota spots in 1942. She was stationed at a Black army field hospital in New Guinea. She remembered caring for a wounded white soldier who was hemorrhaging and close to death. He happened to be closer to the Black hospital than the white one, which was down the river. Burrell and the other Black nurses weren't going to let this man bleed out just because it was against the rules for them to treat white people. But the soldier needed a blood transfusion, and at that time, the Red Cross separated blood donated by Black and white people; mixing the two was not allowed. "We said, 'We're sorry, but the blood is labeled A.' And you know, we knew blood [type] difference in people, yet they had labeled it 'A' for African, their stupid selves. We told him the blood was labeled 'A' so we can't give it, and he said, 'I don't give a damn, don't let me die . . .'" They transfused and stabilized him before he was transferred to the white hospital.

As the war ground on, Staupers leveraged every resource for Black nurses who wanted to serve. She even petitioned the cases of individual nurses to the army and the Red Cross. Louise Virginia Lomax, RN, tried to join the ANC and was also turned away because of her race. Her daughter, Pia Marie Winters Jordan, described what happened: "Evidently, my mother wrote to Mabel Staupers to tell her how hard it was for her to get into the military. Mabel Staupers wrote her a letter back saying, 'We're going to pass this on to the secretary of the army, as another example of discrimination.'" After that, Lomax got one of the quota spots in 1943 and was deployed as a nurse to Tuskegee Air Force Base.

Even as Black nurses tried to volunteer, the parallel narrative emerged that there simply weren't enough nurses to go around. American hospitals couldn't find staff. Nurse shortages were in the headlines during World War II even more than they were in 2020. "Need Emphasized for More Nurses," a 1942 *New York Times* headline proclaimed.

Amid the scarcity, discriminatory and moralizing efforts to define who was a "real" nurse looked increasingly cruel and absurd. In 1942, the ANC suspended its requirement that nurses be unmarried, and it raised the age limit, which had been thirty-five. (But an unmarried pregnancy would still earn you a dishonorable discharge.) Male nurses were not even considered; the ANC was entirely female. In fact, twelve hundred men who happened to be nurses had been drafted, but none of them worked as nurses in the war effort. One, named Jacob Rose, found himself filling potholes in India. Another, Robert Cincotta, wrote to his congresswoman, pointing out that scores of male nurses wanted to volunteer, but were being barred.

In 1943, the army raised its quota for Black nurses from 53 to 160, and then, as the shortage got ever more dire, to about 300 out of a total of about 44,000 in 1944. The small number of Black nurses who were able to join up were often underused, mostly because the army couldn't wrap its head around how to house and feed people together and still maintain segregation. Because of this, at one point, 97 Black nurses were caring for 110 Black servicemen at a base in Arizona while, elsewhere, entire hospitals didn't have a single nurse. At another base in Arizona, Black nurses were relegated to watching over Nazi POWs and saw that the Germans had more perks than they did. The nurses were refused service at restaurants in town, were ignored by white officers on base, and although the POWs had staff to clean their quarters, the nurses did not.

It was an election year, and all over the United States, there was genuine fear that sons would not return home because there would be no one to care for them when they were wounded. The question of nurses became politically charged. Eleanor Roosevelt invited

Staupers to her New York City apartment to discuss the problem. Staupers described for her the plight of Black nurses who were qualified to serve their country in its hour of need, but who were outright denied or relegated to sitting on a base in Arizona, watching over well-fed Nazis. Staupers later wrote that the First Lady "listened and asked the kind of questions that revealed her keen mind and her understanding of the problems." After that, Staupers believed, Eleanor Roosevelt started her own back-channel campaign to remove the restrictions.

But the pivotal moment really came when President Roosevelt started to consider a draft on nurses—which would have been a draft on white women. In January 1945, Norman T. Kirk, who had taken over from Magee as surgeon general of the army, held a meeting in which he announced that a nurse draft might be necessary. Staupers was in that meeting—she seems to have been in every meeting. According to Hine, she jumped up and asked, "If nurses are needed so desperately, why isn't the army using colored nurses?" This tense and awkward moment was covered in newspapers nationwide. It was impossible to deny that Staupers had the moral, patriotic (and logical) upper hand. She quickly organized a campaign that sent a flood of telegrams to the White House, all lamenting the obvious fact that the United States would rather shut out Black nurses than provide adequate care for its soldiers.

That very month, both the army and the navy announced an end to racial quotas, saying both branches would admit female nurses regardless of their race and would not exclude any nurses from serving in any setting. Until that moment, the navy had accepted zero Black nurses. Staupers was, of course, at the meeting in which Rear Admiral William Agnew announced that the navy would drop the color barrier. She pointedly inquired why, if nurses were so badly needed, it was the case that ten days before, Black nurses had been completely barred from the navy. Of course, it was absurd. Agnew could only reply to her plainly that Black nurses would now be accepted.

Staupers was victorious in part because of the very specific moral authority she claimed: she argued that Black nurses, as nurses and as American women, had a responsibility and a right to care for their countrymen. But her victory had implications beyond nursing, and she knew it. Historian Hine writes that Staupers's "effort had culminated in the breaking of at least this one link in the chain which pressed, excluded and prohibited black women from the full realization of their civil rights."

Of course, the fight was not over. Amityville nurse Leftenant-Colon found that even once it was technically possible to sign up, as she did in 1945, she was not exactly welcomed; she likened it to being thrown into a briar patch. At the recruiting office, officials ignored her for as long as they could. "You stood around for a long time because nothing was happening," she remembered seventy-six years later, sitting with her hands neatly clasped. "And that was one way they had of dealing with you: just let you stand around." The armed forces were still segregated, so her status was tenuous. Finally, in 1948, President Truman signed an executive order officially desegregating all the armed forces, and Leftenant-Colon was the first to cross over into the regular Army Nurse Corps, no asterisks. She had already been a nurse for nearly five years and had been serving in the army for three, but the process was arduous. "Take a physical, and an exam. You would think I was being born again," she said.

Leftenant-Colon would go on to be a flight nurse in the Korean War. She flew on transport planes into combat zones, where she picked up badly wounded soldiers and then kept them alive on the flight back to a U.S. base in Japan. She cared for forty to fifty patients per flight, their stretchers stacked like bunks inside the belly of the plane. She was the only nurse on those flights, though she made a point of giving credit to the corpsmen—who could be called nurses, too—who worked with her to care for those injured young men. Leftenant-Colon retired from the military in 1965 with the rank of major. She went on to serve for many years as a public school nurse.

It wasn't until 1955 that the military accepted male nurses, and when it did so, it was again because of another nurse shortage in the armed forces. The Vietnam War loomed, the Cold War smoldered, and a famous incident in which a French nurse got stranded in a battle sparked anxiety over women in combat—and finally, it was agreed that men could nurse for their country. And again, being *allowed* to nurse was very different from being fully *accepted* as a nurse. (The 2000 movie *Meet the Parents* has a running gag based on Ben Stiller's character's being a male nurse and, therefore, hapless and insufficiently masculine.)

Why should everyone care when some nurses are shut out of nursing or told that their nursing is inferior or unreal because of some aspect of their identity? Historian Threat explains it this way: "Nursing is focused on the health of the individual and the community. And if you limit who can support those lofty goals, if you cling to the idea that nurses are women, and often white women, then you are limiting the possibility of every individual and every community to have health." Those stakes could not be higher.

Attempts to limit nursing to certain groups have been damaging and unjust, but they have also never quite worked. When Seacole didn't wait for permission; when Whitman saw the humanity in each broken body; when Taylor, who learned to read in secret, *knew* she was a nurse, not a laundress—all this was nursing in action. And when Staupers harnessed every connection, pressed every case, flew under the twin banners of patriotism and care to break down an edifice of Jim Crow, that was nursing, too.

CHAPTER 4

COMMUNITY

Libraries, Church Basements, and Tenement
Houses: Nursing at Work in Everyday Lives

The white-steepled Seventh Day Adventist church in Benton, Tennessee, sits atop a small rise just off the main road that runs through town. One chilly, blue-sky afternoon in March, signs were posted up the drive, pointing the way to a diabetes seminar. In the church's community hall, long tables were set up and covered with plastic pastel tablecloths. This was the third of eight weekly meetings, and as participants arrived, they chatted and checked their weight and blood pressure before coming into the hall, where church volunteers were handing out small plates of homemade hummus, crackers, and celery. The recipe for the hummus could be found in the participant handbook everyone carried with them.

Stephen Wickham, RN, has the upright bearing of a preacher: tall and thin with a shock of white hair. That day, he wore a tie and a checked shirt, tucked in. Karen Wickham, RN, his wife, stood next to him in a long black-and-red dress. Stephen started the seminar like a religious revival: "Who met their fiber goals this week?" he boomed from the front of the room. A few tentative hands went up. "One! Two! Three!" Stephen said, pointing to each in turn.

"Okay, weight loss! How many met a weight loss goal?" Someone volunteered that they had lost a half pound. "Good! A half pound for you!" he said. "How about walking after meals? Who is walking after meals? One! Two! Three! Four! Very *good*!"

"When you get a diagnosis of diabetes or pre-diabetes, the first thing your physician says is you gotta cut your carbs," said Karen, setting up a slide show on one wall. "But tonight, we're going to explain a little more about carbs. So, sugars, starches, fiber, and cellulose—those are all carbohydrates. All right, here we go!"

Stephen stepped in to explain that many sugars in our food are built with just two simple sugar molecules: glucose and fructose. He said the difference between them is that glucose is a necessary energy source, while fructose can be harmful and, in large amounts, it can be stored as fat in the liver, a factor in diabetes. "You know, these sugars are just like people. They like to reach out and hold hands." He reached for Karen, and the two clasped hands, showing how different sugars are created from those two building blocks and explaining how to spot high-fructose sugars on food packaging.

"But isn't fructose the sweetener in fruit? Does that mean you can't eat fruit anymore?" Stephen asked, then shook his head. "When God packages a toxin in your food supply, he always packages it with the antidote. What do you think the antidote for fructose might be? Fiber, fiber, fiber! Fiber actually undoes everything the sugar's been doing." He pointed out that the amount of fructose in a glass of apple juice is equivalent to eating eight apples at a sitting, a feat most people would not attempt.

"We all love potatoes, right?" Stephen asked the room, which was warming up. He explained that a hot baked potato can spike your blood sugar, but if you bake it, then chill it, the potato undergoes a molecular change to a more resistant starch, which will not spike blood sugar as much. Even better if it's a sweet potato. Same idea for whole grains and whole wheat pasta: "Remember the whole grain pasta salad we had last week?" Karen asked the room. "The ladies cooked the pasta and refrigerated it, and then when you ate it the next evening, it didn't spike your blood sugar."

A church volunteer then led everyone in a series of thirty-second exercise bursts, to show what could be done at home, without equipment: knee raises, arm bends, no-jump jumping jacks. Those who couldn't stand up to do the movements were encouraged to do what they could while seated.

The two-hour session was full of actionable information that could add up to better-controlled type 2 diabetes. The Wickhams run these seminars on a regular basis all over the state of Tennessee. For most people in the room that night, this information was more than they had gotten from their physicians—which was generally a medical model of treatment that could be provided in fifteen-minute visits. They'd been told to drastically cut carbs and lose weight. They'd been prescribed medication to keep symptoms under control for as long as possible. Maybe they had been given a pamphlet with some recipes. For most of them, all this hadn't been enough to stop the deterioration of their health.

The work that the Wickhams do is rooted in their Seventh-day Adventism, a Christian denomination that prioritizes an unprocessed, vegetarian diet. (One of the so-called Blue Zones, where people live much longer than average, is a small community of Adventists in California.) They both grew up with this faith but didn't always follow its dietary tenets—later in life, as nurses, they found it powerful to see that scientific studies confirmed the health value of their beliefs. Most of the participants in their seminars are not Adventists—though

Adventist churches often host the seminars and provide the volunteers. The couple's program contains references to Christian faith alongside evidence-based information, a combination that seems resonant for the communities the Wickhams serve. (The couple also holds seminars in secular spaces, like libraries and city halls across Tennessee.) Their nursing is rooted in a long tradition of community and public health, nursing that takes place outside a hospital or physician's office. It is nursing that meets people where they are and, ideally, provides care in culturally specific ways—at home; at church or synagogue or mandir or mosque; at the library; at homeless shelters; at public schools; and even in grocery stores.

This is a very old kind of nursing, harking back to a time before hospitals were the default, when *most* care happened in the community. Providing care outside the context of acute illness and emergency can be extremely powerful in preventing disease and in changing a wide range of outcomes. For instance, the Nurse-Family Partnership, a venerable program based on forty-five years of research that matches first-time parents with a supportive nurse, has been shown in randomized controlled trials to improve language and behavioral development in children, decrease ER visits, and increase employment for parents. Ideally, this kind of nursing is responsive to a community's specific sources of suffering and desires for care.

The Wickhams designed their program as group sessions located in familiar, easy-to-access locations for a reason: "We need the community involved. You need the social circle if you want that person to be successful," Stephen said. He told me about an inpatient program for people with diabetes, with dietitians on hand and all kinds of classes, but when patients were discharged, they went back to their old habits. "When you bring people into a sterile environment like that, it doesn't work," he said. He points out that physicians often tell patients to lose weight without providing any concrete guidance or support. The message, then, when they don't lose weight or when their diabetes progresses, is that they've failed. "They've heard 'less carbs, less fat.' People don't know how to translate that into specific foods. Calorie restriction will not work. What you need is a program where they can eat ad lib, until they are full." The Wickhams discourage rapid weight loss. Instead, participants in their seminar are guided to set their own goals for fiber intake, exercise, water consumption, and weight loss and to understand the best ways to meet them.

"What we're doing is from a different paradigm," Karen said. Back when they were both nursing in hospitals, Stephen and Karen saw what happened when people with chronic illnesses were unsupported: they just came back, again and again, sicker each time. "Say you're here in the hospital with recurrent pancreatitis," Karen said. "What can you do to prevent coming back to the hospital? I want you to know that *before* you leave." But there's only so much one discharge meeting with a nurse can do about what happens in someone's daily life.

In the Wickhams' experience, almost nothing has brought as much suffering to their community as diabetes. As for many Tennesseans, this is personal for them. Both were pre-diabetic before developing their program by changing their own habits. In 2012, Karen's mother died of diabetes complications.

The idea that type 2 diabetes can be reversed, as the Wickhams say, is new, and the science on it is evolving. (Some existing studies that point to the possibility of reversal have been done by providers who run diabetes reversal clinics and therefore have a conflict of interest.) But there is clear consensus that diabetes remission—a period of at least three months without the aid of medications during which blood glucose levels no longer indicate diabetes—is possible. The difference between reversal and remission seems to be mainly semantic, and proponents of reversal, like the Wickhams, acknowledge that diabetes will return if the new lifestyle habits aren't maintained. The Wickhams know that many or even most of the participants in their seminars will not be able to fully reverse their diabetes, but it's not an all-or-nothing proposition: it's still a victory when people can get their diabetes under better control, reduce reliance on medications, and prevent other cascading problems.

Diabetes is the most expensive chronic disease in the United States—one fourth of all the money spent on health care in the country is spent on diabetes. What are people with diabetes getting for all that money? Diabetes outcomes are only worsening. The fact that lifestyle changes are helpful for some people does not mean that diabetes is a person's fault—diabetes is the result of a complex interplay of genes, environment, behavior, and structural issues. Medication is an important and necessary tool that keeps people alive. But should it be the only tool?

That day in Benton, there were about twenty-eight participants in the room; they were a range of ages, from adolescents to grandmas, and reflective of the surrounding area, which is over 96 percent white, of which a large majority is observantly Christian. Benton, a town of about thirteen hundred people, is in the very southeastern tip of the state, close to both Georgia and North Carolina, a place of rolling blue hills and mountains at the southern end of the Appalachians. The Ocoee River runs through the area, bringing white-water rafting tourism, a major source of employment.

In Polk County, where Benton is the county seat, 15 percent of the population has diabetes, as opposed to about 10 percent in the United States on average. Here, the interlocking root causes are both individual and structural, as they are in many parts of the country, whether urban or rural: relatively low incomes, long or unpredictable work hours. A dearth of fresh produce in local shops leads to a heavily processed diet; the absence of safe sidewalks makes exercise difficult. In Tennessee, nearly two thousand people die of diabetes each year. The people in the church hall had paid forty-five dollars for the eight-session series because they didn't want to become one of those two thousand.

Karen said the most important, overarching element of the program is education: "*Why* they are having these problems. Once they understand why, they intuitively know what to do." The Wickhams' coaching emphasizes three main lifestyle changes: eating lots of fiber, drinking lots of water (no sweetened beverages), and exercising after each meal. (This can be as simple as a walk.) The fiber goals are particularly intense: the Wickhams recommend slowly building up to fifty grams of fiber a day or more. (Most Americans consume only about ten grams a day.) This is *a lot* of fiber. But you can get there in a day by eating, for instance, one cup of raspberries, one pear, one apple, one cup of cooked broccoli, one cup of peas, one cup of lentils, and three cups of air-popped popcorn. (Foods that have no fiber are often animal-based: meats, eggs, cheeses.) It's a neat trick, because piling on the fiber is a simple way to dramatically increase the amounts of fruits, vegetables, beans, and whole grains a person eats, while also improving their gut health, ensuring that they feel full and decreasing blood sugar spikes. Instead of draconian measures that cut out fruits and carbs, the rule is that any carbs or fruit one eats should come with their natural fiber—so fruit juice and refined white flour are discouraged.

These changes are not always accessible, affordable, or easy to sustain, and the Wickhams know this. Stephen often speaks to the managers of small-town local stores about carrying more fruits and vegetables. He said the manager of a particular Save a Lot revamped the entire store to include more fresh produce.

Four years ago, Lee Kent was one of the participants in the Wickhams' diabetes reversal seminar. Kent's father had had diabetes, and even with increasing doses of insulin, it spiraled out of control, until he had to have part of his foot amputated. This can happen when diabetes is not well managed—poor circulation in the hands and feet can result in gangrene or an unhealable wound. Kent's father became increasingly withdrawn. It was devastating for Kent to watch him deteriorate slowly over the course of decades and, finally, to die from complications of the disease.

Years later, when Kent himself was diagnosed with diabetes, he was terrified. By that time, he was on blood pressure and cholesterol medications, and his physician said he would also need to go on metformin to control his blood sugar. Kent already worked out at the gym regularly, despite using a cane, which made high-intensity exercise difficult. He desperately did not want to end up like his dad—he didn't want his children to have to watch him disappear—but he also didn't know how to avoid it. Then a friend at the gym told him about a community-based diabetes reversal program.

Kent remembers his relief when he realized the Wickhams were not just pounding the message that everyone needed to lose an impossible-sounding amount of weight. Instead, they explained how certain changes can make diabetes easier to control and weight easier to lose. They gave out samples of lentil soup and showed participants how to make it using ingredients that could be found in local shops.

Week by week, Kent noticed that his blood sugar numbers were improving. He totally revamped his cooking and even started to like vegetables; before, he didn't really know how to prepare them. He also discovered that he loved chickpeas in all kinds of dishes, and oatmeal with walnuts, apple, and cinnamon. He even passed out once because his blood pressure had dropped so much. His physician took him off all his meds. The sense of progress, the sense of hope, was propulsive for him. "It helped so much being around other people, seeing other people with the same issues as me," Kent says. "It made a total difference in my life."

Now the only thing Kent takes is a multivitamin. He grows and freezes blueberries to snack on all year long. He still enjoys sweets in moderation, but his blood sugar has stayed down. "It's a way of life now," he says, and he credits his survival to the Wickhams. "My kids tell them, 'Thanks for saving my dad's life.'" No one else in the health care system had conveyed any kind of hope to Kent. He had diagnoses and medications, and that was it.

As a country, we seem to just accept things like the cost of insulin rising to three hundred dollars a vial or that people like Kent will die of diabetes. The Wickhams don't accept it, and community health nursing doesn't accept it. Imagine Lee Kent multiplied. Nursing, working in people's *lives*.

Public health or community health nursing is one of the oldest kinds of skilled care. Think of the home visits made by early nurses, midwives, and healers the world over, or of the medieval and early modern convents and monasteries that also functioned as pharmacies and preventative care clinics within their communities. Today, public health nursing and community health nursing overlap, and community health nursing is sometimes thought of as one kind of public health nursing. The distinction between the two often lies in public health's role in big-picture, population-level work, sometimes with governmental agencies—like the response to Covid-19—whereas community health provides direct care to people outside the hospital, care that often includes advocacy and education. A defining quality of this kind of nursing is meeting people where they are, both literally and with regard to their cultural context. And when care leaves the hospital, everything about that care changes—particularly in the degree of autonomy the nurses possess, and in more opportunity for genuine connection between patient and nurse.

Although no single person invented this kind of nursing, the public health nursing movement in the United States was led by a certain woman at a certain time: In 1893, a twenty-six-year-old nurse named Lillian Wald saved a life, and the ripple effects would change the world.

At the time, Wald had recently graduated from the New York Hospital Training School for Nurses, in Manhattan, where she had worked as a trainee in the hospital. Most nights, she had fallen into bed exhausted after a long shift of hustling from one bedside to another. She and the other nurses lived on site, seeing the city only as it manifested in the patients in the hospital beds. Shortly after graduation from the nursing program, she entered medical school. But when friends who worked in philanthropy asked Wald if she would volunteer her nursing skills to help the crowded and desperately poor immigrant communities on the Lower East Side, she realized that she had never given that neighborhood a moment's thought—she knew nothing about the people who lived a ten-minute walk from her dormitory.

Later, she would be embarrassed at the image that came to her mind when she thought of the Lower East Side: "A vague and alarming picture of something strange and alien: a vast crowded area, a foreign city within our own, for whose conditions we had no concern." In response to her friends' request, Wald thought about what she could offer. She proposed a series of classes on home nursing: basic information on hygiene, how to care for a family member at home. She set up a simple classroom in an old building then being used as a technical school. And it was there, on a drizzly, gray morning in March, that everything changed.

Wald was teaching a group of women about bed making—it was not easy to keep anything clean with no plumbing in most tenements—when a little girl burst into the room. Her mother had been bleeding nonstop for two days after giving birth. The family had called a doctor, but he had quickly come and gone after realizing the family couldn't pay. Please, the girl asked, could Wald help?

Wald followed the distraught girl down the unpaved and crowded streets, over dirty mattresses and trash heaps, past tall apartment buildings whose fire escapes teetered with household items. The girl wove through the crowds and open-air fish markets, down Hester Street, to Ludlow Street. Small children played amid the garbage in the gutters, everything damp with rain. Finally, the girl showed Wald into a two-room apartment, which the family of seven shared with several boarders. There, Wald found the girl's mother lying in a bed soaked with her own blood.

Somehow, Wald stopped the bleeding. She stayed until the woman was stable; she cleaned her and made her comfortable. This family had likely never experienced such care—though they *surely* knew women who had died in childbirth in exactly this way—and they were overwhelmed with gratitude. "They kissed my hands," Wald writes. She called it a "baptism of fire."

Wald had grown up in Rochester, New York, the third child in a well-to-do family of German-Jewish origin. Her father sold eyeglasses. Her family was full of scholars, rabbis, and merchants, and her home, while she was growing up, was full of books and music. She was educated at Miss Martha Cruttenden's English-French Boarding and Day School for Young Ladies. Empathy came easily to her, but she had been, by her own account, mostly ignorant of the conditions under which many of her fellow New Yorkers lived.

But when she saved the life of that woman about to bleed to death in her own bed as her children watched, it was a visceral education. That night, Wald lay awake thinking of what she had seen. She thought—naïvely, she said later—that if only people *knew* the conditions of grinding poverty, if only they *knew* how that family lived, those horrors would cease to exist. Now that *she* knew, she could not go on as usual. She realized that, as a nurse, she could be more useful in the city than in a hospital. She turned this idea over and over in her mind. Later, she described this, and everything that came next, in a book called *The House on Henry Street*.

The next morning, she poured out the story to a friend. As she spoke, she found herself presenting a plan, without having really meant to: she would live on the Lower East Side, and she would offer nursing care to the people in the neighborhood. It was both a great idea and an incredibly unlikely plan for an upper-class unmarried woman at the time. But Wald would never return to hospital work, nor to the expectations others had for her. She described the beginning of her new life this way: "Within a day or two, a comrade from the training school, Mary Brewster, agreed to share in the venture. We were to live in the neighborhood as nurses, identify ourselves with it socially, and in brief, contribute to it our citizenship."

Wald and Brewster found themselves a top-floor apartment in a tenement building on Jefferson Street that had the rarest of amenities: an indoor bathroom. (Wald writes, "According to legend at the time there were only two bathrooms in tenement houses below Fourteenth Street.") They could open the windows for fresh air and were delighted to have access to the roof through the fire escape. They decorated the place with interesting bits of copper and brass they bought from a man under the elevated subway on Allen Street.

When word spread that two nurses were providing services on a pay-what-you-can basis, Brewster and Wald became busy from morning to night, visiting sick neighbors and grappling with the daily problems of poverty. People often showed up at their door first thing in the morning. All this was exactly as Wald had envisioned it.

As a clinician, Wald did not hold herself apart from her neighbors. Instead, she invited their children to dinner. In fact, she loved living on the Lower East Side, even as she recognized that the unjust conditions there were killing people. "The mere fact of living in the tenement brought undreamed-of opportunities for widening our knowledge and extending our human relationships," she writes. When winter fell, it brought a brutal economic depression and dangerous cold. Wald and Brewster lugged their nursing bags from walk-up to walk-up from sunup to sundown.

This was a very particular moment on the Lower East Side. Thousands of people were arriving on boats every day, mainly from Russia and Italy, and there was no assistance whatsoever to help them get started in this new country—no housing or workplace regulations, no restrictions on child labor, no food safety regulations or food stamps, no public housing, no Medicaid. The Lower East Side was said to be the most crowded place in the world. One square block was home to 2,800 people. (Today it is less than half as dense.) When horses died in the street, they lay where they fell. Children played in the gutter near dead animals and running sewage. The drinking water was rarely clean, and infections spread quickly. Devastating fires were common. Twenty-seven percent of babies living in the neighborhood died before their first birthday.

Wald was radicalized by her neighbors' sorrow. One nearby family desperately wanted to keep the tradition of a Friday Shabbat dinner but had no food. They kept two large pots bubbling over the fire, but there was only water inside. Another family had no furniture because they had burnt it all to keep from freezing to death. One of their children had died anyway and, because the family had no money, had been buried in a mass public grave. The family kept trying to scrape together the money to have their child's body disinterred and buried in a consecrated grave, but each time they accumulated any savings, they instead gave the money to neighbors down the hall, to keep their children from starving. Many of Wald's immigrant neighbors were religiously observant Jewish or Catholic, and their shared circumstances often superseded cultural or language differences: Wald writes of the time an Orthodox Jewish woman who had been on her knees scrubbing floors all day walked many extra blocks to ask Wald to get a priest for her neighbors' dying child.

In 1895, Wald and Brewster decided they needed more space and a more organized approach to their nursing service. They moved to a row house on nearby Henry Street, purchased and renovated as a gift from Wald's friend, banker philanthropist Jacob Schiff. There they established a "nurse's settlement," a permanent home where nurses could live and provide care for neighbors. This eventually became the United States' first official visiting nurse service. Wald referred to the working community of women who lived at Henry Street as "the family." It was a place of rare female autonomy, a close support system outside the bounds of the era's typical family life. (Wald had romantic relationships with two of the women.)

These social service–oriented, progress-minded settlement houses existed elsewhere—such as Jane Addams's Hull House in Chicago—but when other settlements provided nursing, they often did so at an on-site clinic. Visiting nursing was fundamentally different. It didn't require a sick person to get out of bed, or to get off work, or to figure out what to do with their children in order to visit a clinic. It inverted the power dynamic. And when nurses visited a home, they could better figure out what the family's larger needs were: Did they have heat, did they have food? Did the children have clothes?

Wald and Brewster—and, later, their many colleagues—provided care where there had been none. At the time, there was no health insurance, and most physicians charged high fees for their services. Private one-on-one nursing was also available—but, again, only for those who could afford it. Some free nursing was available through various religious organizations, but only to members. Several city hospitals, like Bellevue, provided care for free to impoverished people, but these were often not people's first choice if they could help it. Wald dexterously cultivated close relationships with New York philanthropists like Schiff so she could offer a flexible pay-if-you-can model. She did not want her nursing service to hinge on affiliation with a physician or a religion, and she was determined that the nursing she provided be "on terms most considerate of the dignity and independence of patients." She developed this model more than one hundred years ago, and it is still completely radical in its insistence on the autonomy and inherent dignity of all people.

When there was a physician involved in a case, Wald and Brewster were obliged to work with him. And even though Wald herself had completed a few years of medical school, one of a small number of women to do so, she and Brewster had to be careful not to seem to overstep. Wald knew of more than one woman left to hemorrhage to death in childbirth when she couldn't pay a physician. Wald assumed that physicians would *want* to disavow any colleagues who did this, but when she brought the situation to their attention, she was met with "the stone wall of professional etiquette." So, she did what she could, working closely with the physicians who were helpful and around the ones who were not.

In 1906, Wald hired Elizabeth Tyler, a Black nurse who had graduated from the Freedmen's Hospital Training School for Nurses, in Washington, DC. Wald would eventually hire twenty-five Black nurses in all, paying them all the same wage and referring to them with the same titles of respect she used with the white nurses. But she could not find patients for them in the neighborhood. Henry Street Settlement itself was not segregated, but much of health care was, and white families would turn away a Black nurse who appeared at their door.

Tyler had the idea to open a branch of Henry Street uptown, in San Juan Hill, a neighborhood on the West Side, near what would one day become Lincoln Center. It was then a poor area with a large Black community. Wald got funding for a building on West Sixty-Second Street, called Stillman House, where Tyler, Edith Carter, Emma Wilson, and other Black nurses lived and provided care. Tyler started out by befriending the janitors of the nearby buildings, who knew everything about everyone, a tactic Wald had also used. Stillman House would eventually provide not just nursing care but also services like banking; classes in dancing, carpentry, and sewing; a playground; and a traveling branch of the New York Public Library.

By 1907, there were ten branches of the settlement all around the city, and the *New York Times* covered Wald's nurses with admiration: "They are highly organized without being institutional, a combination hard to find. They radiate neighborly help, not red-taped formal assistance but just plain, natural, capable help."

As chronicled in the *Times*, a day in the life of an unnamed Henry Street nurse looked like this: In the morning, it was off to a canal boat on one of the rivers, where someone had pneumonia. The nurse climbed over and through several boats to reach the patient's vessel. From there, she went to check on a mother and her newborn baby; the woman's husband has just died, leaving her destitute. Next, the nurse went to see about an old man's injured leg; the man wanted a little gossip along with the bandage. Then she stopped at the apartment of an Irish woman and her son. The woman was disabled but managed at home with the daily household help of the nurse. Then, to an Italian household where the father of the family was dying. The wife wanted to care for her husband, but she was a garment worker and was occupied sewing piecework nonstop all day. The nurse made the dying man more comfortable and left, still thinking about the family. After a quick lunch, she went back to the man with pneumonia on the canal boat; she was not encouraged by his condition. Then she was off to see a little girl who was recovering from an illness, to explain a change in medication to the girl's mother; she brought some flowers for the girl. Finally, she was back on the river, in the canal boat again; the patient had not improved. She made a telephone call to update the night nurse, who would be caring for him on the next shift. On the way home, she had an idea: she could use Henry Street funds to hire someone to do the Italian woman's daily sewing for a while, so that the woman could spend her time with her husband and still keep her job.

By 1914, Wald employed at least ninety-two nurses, who cared for thousands of people, making two hundred thousand visits each year all over Manhattan and the Bronx. Only about 10 percent of the Henry Street patients ended up having to be admitted to the hospital. Public health nursing worked, and Wald was able to prove it.

In those days, before antibiotics, children died of infections that are routine for us now. Wald tracked pneumonia outcomes for children under two, the most likely to die. In 1914, 9 percent of these children died under the care of a visiting nurse. By comparison, in the four largest hospitals in New York City, the same group with the same illness died an average of 38 percent of the time; at one hospital, it was 51 percent.

Much of nursing's power lies in the one-on-one relationship with a patient, but many of the root causes of illnesses are bigger social problems that can't be solved individually. Public health nursing, as Wald conceived it, seeks to address these larger conditions: Some of the most important societal advances of the twentieth century came directly out of her nursing insights.

Even a partial list of her achievements is so long as to be almost absurd: Wald spearheaded the country's first public municipal playground—first, in the backyard at Henry Street and, then, the one still in operation at Seward Park in Manhattan—so that children could play somewhere safe. (She said children's play was a matter of "dignity.") Seeing that illnesses spread at school and then kept children out of school, she proposed the concept of the school nurse, and Henry Street paid the salary of the first school nurse for a year, which led the city to adopt the idea in 1902. She also pressured the public schools to start providing lunch. She and a Henry Street teacher developed the first model of special education, funded a pilot program, and then urged the Board of Education to adopt it citywide. By 1915, three thousand disabled children benefited from specially trained teachers. She also helped to establish the federal Children's Bureau and to outlaw child labor. She was a co-chair of the American Union Against Militarism, a pacifist organization founded in response to World War I. Because she thought the arts were not just for the rich or the assimilated, she also funded Yiddish theater and children's music programs. And she hosted W. E. B. Du Bois, Ida B. Wells, and others at Henry Street for the conference in which the National Association for the Advancement of Colored People (NAACP) was founded. She saw that all these efforts were connected and that all of them were within the purview of nursing.

How did she do all this? She was a natural collaborator. And she was a kind of evangelist, both a true believer and a pragmatist who nimbly navigated the city's many worlds. She was the only radical socialist who was always invited to dinner by wealthy New York society. She never came right out and asked for donations, but she parted the rich from their money with charming or heart-tugging anecdotes about the need for more nurses—rueful word went around high society that sitting next to Wald at dinner would cost you five thousand dollars—and she kept the humanity of all involved at the very center of what she did.

She always focused on people more than policy: In describing the importance of special education, she told the story of a boy named Tony, who came from Naples. In first grade, Tony's teachers gave up on him—he often had disruptive outbursts in class and was frequently absent. At a special education class at Henry Street, it turned out that he needed glasses and that working with his hands helped him focus. Tony grew up to be a union bricklayer and was able to buy a house for his family in Brooklyn.

Wald lived and worked as a nurse on the Lower East Side for forty years, until she retired from the Henry Street Settlement in 1933. She died several years later, at the age of seventy-three. Today, the neighborhood is much changed, but the Henry Street Settlement is still there, in the original row house, plus the two adjoining, which were added in subsequent years. New York City neighbors still use the programs to find safe and clean housing, affordable health care on a sliding scale, jobs, English-language training, arts, and children's programs. (Visiting Nurse Service of New York, also Wald's creation, branched off from the Henry Street Settlement years ago.)

Curious visitors can take a tour of the original Henry Street house, all creaky wood and narrow staircases. Wald's bedroom, with a fireplace and a large balcony overlooking the backyard, where children played and labor leaders met, has been made into a meeting room. The narrow nurses' bedrooms are now program offices. Outside, a red banner hangs, printed in English, Chinese, and Spanish: WE ARE HERE TO HELP! BENEFITS/SNAP, LEGAL AND FINANCIAL SERVICES, AFFORDABLE HEALTH INSURANCE, PARENT CENTER.

Organizations for visiting nurses still exist, of course—when my daughter, Mira, came home from the hospital, it was a visiting nurse, prescribed by the discharging physicians, who came and weighed her and made sure she was stable her first two weeks living at home. That nurse's daily visits were my lifeline; she helped me see the other side of the sleepless, fearful time I was living in then. But when your kid has an ear infection, or your elderly mother needs a vaccine, or you need a nurse to help you manage your diabetes—that is now generally done in a physician's office, hospitals, or urgent care locations, not at home.

The fact that visiting and community health nursing did not become as prevalent as one might think has a lot to do with a huge change in the ways Americans die and in the profit motivations that followed. In the early decades of the twentieth century, the Metropolitan Life Insurance agency partnered with Wald to offer visiting nursing to their policyholders. The logic was that if these nurses could prevent premature deaths, life insurance agencies could make fewer early payouts and be more profitable. At first, this worked well for everyone, and Metropolitan Life contracted with visiting nurse agencies in several large cities, to care for policyholders when they were ill. Visiting nursing was expanding.

But as the years ticked by, the advent of antibiotics and vaccines meant that many fewer people were dying prematurely of fast-moving, acute infectious diseases. Now people were living longer, but they were also living for years with chronic illnesses like diabetes and heart disease. Those conditions didn't kill them quickly, but they were also not curable and necessitated *years* of nursing care, not weeks. If a nurse provides two weeks of intensive home nursing to prevent a forty-year-old person from dying of pneumonia, and if that forty-year-old goes on to live twenty-five more years, that's a great deal from a life insurance company's point of view. If a nurse spends the last five years of an elderly person's life helping them more comfortably manage their diabetes at home, and if they die around the age they would have anyway, that is a terrible financial deal for the life insurance company. Nurses, left to their own devices in people's homes, tended to put the patients' needs above concerns about cost. Meanwhile, the hospital became more central to all kinds of care, especially with the advent of health insurance. It was an entirely different model, one that did not prioritize the relationship between nurse and patient.

Visiting nursing was very popular with patients. In 1947, Metropolitan Life's own research bureau found that there was still large potential demand for home nursing and that people who received this care were almost universally happy with it. But it was no longer cost-effective for MetLife, so the company ended the program. Now roughly 60 percent of all registered nurses work in inpatient hospitals, and hospitals are seen as the default setting for nurse practice. Urgent cares can fill in some of these clinical gaps, but react to problems rather than prevent them, and their model doesn't allow for building therapeutic relationships or following a patient for the long-term. The immense potential good of community health nursing has yet to be realized.

Still, community health nursing persists in schools, in community centers, and even at Walmart. In Pima, Arizona, for instance, public health nurses offer basic services at the library, where they do blood pressure screenings, answer questions, and make referrals. By working at the library, they reach a broad swath of the community, from parents of young children to people experiencing homelessness.

Crucially, when nurses are rooted in a community, they can identify and respond to a problem faster and more effectively than those on the outside. In some cases, like a disease outbreak, the quick mobilization of nurses can save lives and prevent a broader epidemic. In New York City, for instance, a tenacious group of Jewish nurses were among the only health care providers who could effectively reach the large ultra-Orthodox Jewish communities in Brooklyn during a recent measles flare-up.

In the fall of 2018, it became evident to Tobi Ash, BSN, RN, and her colleagues in the Orthodox Jewish Nurses Association that something was going very wrong. According to data shared by city and state health departments, measles cases in ultra-Orthodox communities in New York and New Jersey were ticking up quickly. Measles is one of the world's most contagious diseases; if an infected person coughs in a room and then leaves, an unvaccinated person can catch measles just by breathing inside that room as much as two hours later. This was particularly relevant in ultra-Orthodox communities: Families there often have many children, and in New York City particularly, living spaces are tight. Extended families might eat dinner together, and men often go to synagogue together twice a day. Before anyone knew what was going on, the number of cases of easy-to-spread measles went from a handful to hundreds. Ash remembered that, at some point, she and her colleagues realized that the case numbers should have been impossible—the only way measles could spread in this way was if people had stopped getting vaccinated against it.

Ash was born and raised in an ultra-Orthodox Hasidic community in Brooklyn, the daughter, granddaughter, and great-granddaughter of prominent rabbis. She has been a nurse since the 1990s, and she splits her time between New York and Miami, where she provides health education at Jewish schools and works as the director of women's health at a clinic. She no longer lives in a Hasidic community, but she has close personal ties there and remains Orthodox.

As the measles outbreak accelerated, Ash and her colleagues realized they had to reach the young women. It was mothers who were making the vaccination decisions for their children, but they were receiving anti-vaccination misinformation from people Ash describes as "nocters": health coaches, chiropractors, and naturopaths, whom the Orthodox community often trusted more than their regular pediatricians. Similar anti-vaccine propaganda, from outsiders like Robert

Kennedy Jr., also found a foothold. People were passing around a booklet called *PEACH* (short for *Parents Educating and Advocating for Children's Health*), which spread fear about autism and discouraged mothers from vaccinating their children. In a community that was often marginalized and scapegoated, many with family members who had suffered through or perished in the Holocaust, it was not hard to believe that vaccines could be harmful—that there were nefarious forces out there wanting to hurt their children.

The city government was trying to reach the community to encourage vaccination, but its tactics were often culturally inept and only sowed more distrust. When the messaging was written in Yiddish, it often read as if it had been run through Google Translate. (Ash says that, in more recent years, the city has much improved its Yiddish outreach.)

In response, several nurses got together to form the EMES (Yiddish for "truth") Initiative to reach these mothers and to counteract the anti-vaccine propaganda that was sending scores of children to the hospital with the infection's characteristic painful rash, high fever, and barking cough. The group leveraged its place in the community as Jewish women and trained nurses not associated with Big Pharma or the government. They arranged comfortable group meetings in people's living rooms, where they listened to mothers' questions and fears and conveyed accurate information on vaccines.

Ash and her colleagues didn't drown the participants in statistics. Instead, they approached these mothers with no judgment and with the understanding that they were just trying to protect their children. "Belief systems are incredibly complex, and they can't be dismantled with information," Ash said. "If this is your belief system, all the logic and proof in the world is never, ever, ever going to make you say, 'Oh my God, I never thought of that.' So, emotion has to be fought with emotion."

And in this case, the nurses' emotion was based in empathy: *I care about you. I understand your family. Please talk to me about your worries.* The women brought up a range of concerns, and the nurses listened and responded. Some women thought that pediatricians were exceedingly rich because the pharmaceutical companies were paying them to push vaccines. The nurses pointed out that pediatricians in the area made much less than the mothers imagined and that it is usually health insurance companies, which have a financial interest in preventing disease, that pay physicians.

The EMES nurses tailored their outreach to the community. They started having larger, more elaborate meetings, with raffles and hot food provided. They noticed that young ultra-Orthodox women were often on Instagram, so they engaged on that platform. And Ash and several others wrote a rebuttal to *PEACH*, in the form of a vaccine safety handbook puckishly titled *PIE* (for *Parents Informed and Educated*). They decided on a physical book because, on Shabbat, ultra-Orthodox people don't use electricity and often spend time reading.

In the end, 1,282 cases of measles resulted from the outbreak, leading to more than 100 hospitalizations in New York City—all from a disease that had been eliminated in the United States. But there likely would have been even more without the efforts of the EMES nurses—and their work is ongoing. Wald would have recognized their framework. It's not about cases or policy; it's about people.

Back in Tennessee, when the presentation portion of the Wickhams' seminar was over, participants broke up into small groups to check in on personal goals and plan high-fiber meals for the week. The facilitator was a church volunteer, an older woman with a dark bob and a kind face; coincidentally, she was a retired nurse. "What's been the hardest thing so far?" she asked the group, which consisted of two men and a woman with her grandson.

The woman brandished her large plastic cup of soda, which she had brought in. "I've got to give this up. I can't. It's the worst." She'd never found it easy to drink water.

The group talked about strategies: Drink a lot of water right when you wake up, or drink it very cold, to cut cravings for other beverages. One of the men said he understood he should eat fruits and vegetables, but he said he found it hard to figure out how to "get the foods together," that is, what dishes to prepare. The other man volunteered that he had been making a smoothie of unsweetened almond milk, oatmeal, quinoa, banana, and apple. There was a country store across the street, and the woman suggested everyone try the oranges there. "Best oranges I ever had in my life." Stephen Wickham, upon hearing the conversation, came over to suggest a few recipe websites. The facilitator asked how everyone liked the hummus; no one really did. "When would you eat that?" one of the men asked. The woman said that her healthy-eating sister-in-law made it for a movie snack.

There were no easy fixes in the room, but there was new information and a lot of ideas—and something else, too: a sense of their all being in this together. They'd do their best this week. They'd come back next week. They'd try again.

CHAPTER 5

ENDINGS

Nursing Beyond Cures: The Radical
Promise of Hospice

On a cold morning in January, Mariana Sandarovscaia, CHPN, RN, was looking for parking in Brighton, a neighborhood in Boston. She made a U-turn into a spot and then reached into the backseat to gather a few items sealed in sterile packets: a new foley catheter, a catheter insertion tray, and a catheter drainage bag. She then fitted an N95 mask onto her face. Her patient's wife met us at the door of their building, and we took an old elevator up to the fourth floor and entered a cozy apartment with white stucco walls and lots of books. Sandarovscaia's patient, whom I'll call Ahmad, was seated upright in bed, covered with a fluffy white duvet and wearing a brown-and-cream striped sweater.

Sandarovscaia and Ahmad greeted each other warmly. Ahmad was eighty-five years old, a creative writing professor emeritus with a handsome, angular, bespectacled face. He had thought he was going to die a year before. That was when he declined surgical treatment for a prostate abscess that didn't respond to intravenous antibiotics. He developed sepsis, and the infection spread to his blood. Invasive surgery to remove the abscess was the last option, but he didn't want a painful, risky procedure; he wanted to go home. He was discharged with home nursing from Good Shepherd Community Care, an extraordinary, nurse-led hospice based nearby, in Newton. Founded in the 1970s, it is committed to the original, revolutionary model of modern nurse-led hospice care.

To everyone's surprise, including his own, Ahmad didn't die. "You die of sepsis quite fast, like within days," said Sandarovscaia. "But he's actually stabilized, and now the more pronounced symptoms are cardiac." What Ahmad thought would be a quick decline and death turned into a slow and mostly gentle one, leaving him time to be with his wife and to read. But his symptoms were sometimes disturbing: he had atrial fibrillation, a dangerous heart arrhythmia also known as A-fib, and his heart rate sometimes roller-coastered from forty to two hundred beats per minute. Unable to urinate, he used a foley catheter and sometimes had the uncomfortable feeling that he needed to pee but couldn't. He often found himself on the verge of fainting when he tried to walk.

Sandarovscaia said it was hard to know his exact prognosis, because the cardiac issues were unpredictable. "He could have an event and die today," she said. "With his symptoms, I would say he would have six months or less. But he has a supportive wife and great quality of care at home. If his heart is able to, there are reasons for him to stay longer. He said that his father and brother died of a heart attack. So, this is his wish: quick and without pain, without prolonging the suffering. I am hoping that this will happen."

When Sandarovscaia arrived that day, Ahmad looked thin and frail; his shortness of breath was audible—quick huffs from under his mask—but he also seemed content sitting in his simple, windowed room. He had books within reach, an adjustable reading lamp, and a shelf stocked with medications, clean towels, and a small vase of wildflowers. Sandarovscaia silently noted details as she walked in: how Ahmad was dressed; the expression on his wife's face; Ahmad's posture in the bed. She noticed that he had fresh drinking water and a small brass bell on the caddy by the bed. There was nothing on the floor around the bed that might cause him to trip when he got up. Sandarovscaia's care always begins with noticing, before conversation, before she lays hands on a patient.

As she always does, she took off her coat, to show there was no hurry, and sat down so that she was eye level with Ahmad, not hovering over him. Then they talked. On each visit, for about an hour, she chats with Ahmad and his wife, asking about his symptoms, gauging their emotional states and their understanding of the situation. She adjusts medications if necessary. The hospice has two physicians on staff who write orders for medications quite broadly: for instance, between five and twenty milligrams of morphine as often as every hour, five milligrams for mild pain, twenty for severe pain. This gives nurses significant flexibility to use their own judgment based on what a patient is experiencing. It also gives control back to the patient, to gauge their own pain level and use the medications as they see fit. Being ill and hospitalized deprives people of agency, and when someone leaves the hospital to enter hospice care, Sandarovscaia aims to empower them. "As long as it's not detrimental, I want them to feel in control of their decisions. And to trust us," she said. She does more listening than talking: "I had an instructor in school who said there is a reason we have two ears and only one mouth."

At first, Ahmad was reluctant to take medications that might change his mental state—many hospice patients are—but with Sandarovscaia's encouragement, he came to find that morphine (for shortness of breath) and lorazepam (for panic and sleeplessness) made him feel better. And feeling better was the *entire* goal. Sandarovscaia made sure the medicines were within his reach even before he was ready to try them. Uncontrolled pain is anathema to hospice care. (Good Shepherd has solutions for families with substance use disorders, like lockboxes. Sometimes a nurse goes every day to deliver medications if it's not safe to leave more than a day's supply with a patient.) Part of Good Shepherd's strategy is to anticipate every need before it arises so that there's never a moment of panic if pain or shortness of breath or delirium starts to spiral out of control. Instead, everything a patient needs is already in place so there can be ease and a sense of normalcy, even though, of course, it's everyone's first time dying.

Sandarovscaia asked Ahmad how his symptoms had been since she saw him last. He said he hadn't had a cardiac episode that day, but that he had had a frightening one the day before. He described it professorially and from a second-person remove. "The heart suddenly from nowhere starts a palpitation. If you look at your chest, you can visually see it, the ribs and the chest," he said, cupping his rib cage to show the movement. "With that goes this feeling in the whole bones of the face and the skull and the jaws and the teeth; they sort of heat up, quite like pain. Not quite pain, but the two together are very unpleasant."

"Like a tension pain?" Sandarovscaia asked. "Yes," he said. She asked how long it lasted, and he replied that, sometimes, if he lay down and rested, it would go away. But sometimes it continued, and with it came shortness of breath. It was then that he would take the morphine and, if it was night, the lorazepam also. Sandarovscaia asked if this happened even when he was resting in bed, and he nodded. They talked about an earlier incident, when he nearly fainted in the bathroom but didn't call for help because he didn't want to worry his wife. Sandarovscaia reminded him to be careful to use his walker when standing and moving around, so as not to fall. Earlier, she got him a special walker with a seat, so that now he can sit down immediately if he feels faint.

Describing these cardiac episodes, Ahmad said that just knowing what to do was enormously reassuring. When he woke in the night gasping for air, he knew which medications to take; they were waiting for him in pre-measured syringes. He wondered if he would die, but he didn't have to wonder what to do. In this sense, he explained to me, dying can be like driving a car: your body knows what to do, so you relax. Sandarovscaia had mentioned earlier that a big part of her job was gentle teaching. She was preparing Ahmad for a journey he had to take alone, but it was a journey she'd seen people take many times. By explaining what to do and when, making sure he had everything he needed to be comfortable, she took away a lot of his fear.

A month or two before, Ahmad's urinary catheter had started to leak. "My wife got very panicked and scared," he said. "She wanted to do something, but she didn't know what to do. She called Mariana on the phone. My wife was talking to her and was crying. After the conversation was over, with more than the speed of an ambulance, Mariana was here. I don't know how she did it and where she found parking! The presence of her—this empathy—somehow comforted my wife, and then comforting *her* comforted *me*." One tenet of hospice is that the family and loved ones are being cared for alongside the person who is dying.

Sandarovscaia confirmed with Ahmad that, for now, his symptoms were well controlled with the existing medications. She replaced the drainage bag from the urinary catheter, listened to his lungs, checked his blood oxygenation with an oximeter, and then read his blood pressure. As the cuff squeezed his wrist, he looked out a window at the gray winter sky and bare treetops. "A dry tree with no leaves against the sky. It's so beautiful, you know," he said, almost to himself. His blood pressure was high, 200 over 113. "I see this is high; let's do it again," Sandarovscaia said calmly. "Are you having any headaches?" She checked back over the blood pressure numbers that Ahmad had recorded himself earlier in the week; they ranged from normal to high. She was satisfied, at least, that there was nothing that needed to be done differently now. The visit over, Sandarovscaia reminded Ahmad and his wife to call her anytime.

We headed back out to the car to go to the next visit. Sandarovscaia's long blonde hair was pulled back tightly into a ponytail, and she wore two layers of fuzzy sweaters with jeans and boots. She grew up in Moldova when it was part of the Soviet Union, and she ascribes her comfort with emotional heaviness to her background. "I don't allow myself to lose my composure in front of patients, but I allow myself when I'm in the car or at home to talk about my feelings. I was raised with the idea that life is hard. But, yes, sometimes I cry. And then I'm so glad I can see the sunset. I have to enjoy it. Not *for* them, but just," she paused, thought. "To keep going."

Several years ago, Sandarovscaia was working as a bedside nurse at a rehabilitation facility when Natalia Khalaydovsky, RN, from Good Shepherd, was assigned to provide hospice for one of Sandarovscaia's patients. (Hospice nurses can provide care in facilities or in homes.) The patient was an elderly woman who had stopped eating and drinking. Within a medical model, when a patient stops eating and drinking, there is an emphasis on finding a fix, such as the insertion of a feeding tube. The tube can go through the nose to the stomach or can be surgically inserted directly into the abdomen. But for people approaching the end of life, often there's no real benefit to be gained from these procedures, which are invasive and uncomfortable. The person will die soon anyway.

"I had this ethical dilemma," Sandarovscaia said. "My patient didn't *want* to eat or drink, but our focus was 'Nutrition is so important. You have to eat; you have to drink.' But when you are not able to, it's very upsetting and also upsetting to the family." When hospice got involved, all this changed. Sandarovscaia was given permission to care for the patient in a way that felt right; in fact, it felt revolutionary to follow the patient's lead. Khalaydovsky told her not to worry about quantifying the patient's intake and, instead, to redefine success as whatever the patient wanted and could tolerate. "That was all new to me," Sandarovscaia said. "Help this patient to be comfortable." Later, Khalaydovsky suggested that Sandarovscaia apply for a job at Good Shepherd, and so she did—and got it.

That was four years ago. Now, driving to our next appointment with classical music on the radio, Sandarovscaia told me about how she navigated emotionally charged situations in which a patient's family or the patient (or both) did not accept that the end was approaching, even though the patient had entered hospice care. To have hospice covered by insurance, patients must generally give up coverage for curative treatment. This means a cancer patient will no longer get chemotherapy but will be treated for symptoms. It can be very difficult for patients and families to accept palliative instead of curative care. (Hospice care is comprehensive care for those who will likely die within six months. Palliative care is focused on comfort, not cure. Palliative care is part of hospice, but palliative care can also be provided in other contexts, whether someone will die soon or not.) Sandarovscaia isn't interested in pushing anyone. She pointed out that hospice is not a contract; people in it can always change their minds. She says she often engages in subtle prompting, trying to help patients adjust to this sad, new world where cures are not possible and are no longer the goal.

Accordingly, one of Sandarovscaia's primary goals is to prevent unnecessary hospitalizations—like a family member panicking and calling 911, for instance, when there is nothing productive that an emergency department can do. She said that some families still fight, within themselves and with one another, over the process. Grief sometimes comes with refusal: an insistent *no*. Sandarovscaia has to be comfortable with that no, which can manifest itself in all kinds of ways. She has to be willing to wade in. Her work is not *just* about dosing medicines, or preventing pressure sores, or making sure someone has the right walker. Each time she visits a patient, she has to marshal her best self to be with the patients as they are. She does this in service of the care, in order to soothe what the founder of modern hospice memorably termed "total pain."

The modern hospice movement was developed in reaction to the development of modern medicine, and its physician-led emphasis on technological advancements and cures—which are, in many ways, miracles but which cannot, in the end, prevent death. In earlier times, most deaths occurred at home, with family or sometimes nurses present. Or end-of-life care was carried out in monasteries or hospitals by nuns and monks, whose spiritual careers required a certain comfort level with death. But in the early- to mid-twentieth century, as medicine became more complex and technological—more able to cure—the meaning of end-of-life care started to change. More sick people spent more time in hospitals, and not all of them could be cured. But in a culture of medical progress, death was seen as a failure, and dying people were often ignored. Later, with the advent of intensive care, people could spend their last days being kept "alive," but without any of the benefits of being alive. In hospital paternalism, in which the doctor was always right, a dying person's wishes, fulfillment, comfort, and even their right to know their diagnosis or prognosis, were not always honored.

One nurse spent her life fighting to establish a better way. Cicely Saunders was born in 1918, the eldest child in a well-off London family. She was a shy girl who often felt like an outsider. As a young woman, she became a nurse, a vocation she felt called to despite the disapproval of her family. But she struggled with the physical demands of the job because of a painful spinal disorder and was "invalided out" of nursing. So, she went back to school for public administration and then began work as what was called a lady almoner, a kind of medical social worker.

In 1947, working at Highgate's Archway Hospital, she met David Tasma, a forty-year-old Polish Jewish man who was dying of advanced rectal cancer with unmanaged pain and vomiting. What we know of Tasma's life is harrowing. He had escaped from the Warsaw Ghetto and fled to London, where he worked as a waiter, only to find himself dying young of a terrible cancer. When Saunders met Tasma, he was completely alone, waiting for death and feeling that his life had been meaningless. Over weeks and months, she visited with him each day, and the two developed a loving friendship—an ambiguous but intense relationship complicated by his terminal illness. They often discussed what real comfort in dying might be like and how different that would be from what he and others were experiencing at the time. His pain—physical, existential, emotional—changed the course of Saunders's life and of history.

Their intimacy gave her an understanding of what she would come to call "total pain," a combination of the physical symptoms, mental distress, social problems, and spiritual needs that come with dying. All around her, she saw that most aspects of that total pain went completely untreated. Physicians were worried about the addictive qualities of opioids and doled them out sparingly, often requiring that one dose wear off before they gave another, instead of administering doses on a schedule that would prevent breakthrough pain. Dying patients were told there was nothing to be done, and often, they were simply left alone. In hospitals, they were no one's priority. Families of the dying often had to abide by restrictive visiting hours, and people died suffering and alone without being able to say good-bye to loved ones.

When Tasma died, he left Saunders everything he had: five hundred British pounds from life insurance (nearly twenty thousand pounds today), his watch, and photographs. In return, he had one request: that she open a home dedicated to caring for the dying and "Let me be a window in your home." It was an enigmatic directive, at least on the face of it, but Saunders would make it literal.

First, she went back to school to become a physician. She saw physicians as one major source of the problem of desertion of the dying but also as the potential solution. Physicians, she felt, were the ones with the power to transform end-of-life care, and because she wanted to change how pain was managed, she had to be able to prescribe medicines. In short, she became a physician to bring her nursing insight into medicine. Nineteen years later, in 1967, with the help of the money Tasma had left her, she opened the first modern in-patient hospice, St Christopher's Hospice. It would not only provide direct care, but would also spark a wider movement, by defining and advocating hospice care.

Saunders, a religious Anglican, named the hospice after the patron saint of travelers, though it was always open to those of all faiths or none. The idea that a hospice is for travelers is an evocative metaphor, but it also has a historically literal meaning. The word *hospice* comes from the Latin *hospitium*—the English words *hospitality* and *hospital* also flow from the same word. In the European Middle Ages, a hospice was a refuge for travelers, sometimes Crusaders, who were sick or dying or who just needed rest, and they usually were run by monks or nuns. The Italian monk Camillus de Lellis, born in 1550, founded one of the first organized hospice programs in Europe. De Lellis came to the work when he went to San Giacomo degli Incurabili, a hospital in Rome, seeking treatment for a leg wound. He never fully recovered his own health, but became a nurse at the hospital. He believed that nursing was an expression of love, and it bothered him that many dying people never got any care at all, especially those who were poor or far from home. So, he founded an order of monk-nurses called the Fathers of a Good Death which nursed dying people at home or would pay innkeepers to allow them the use of their rooms for this purpose.

Saunders was very aware of this history. "Hospice is about a special kind of living and, in a sense, is still concerned with traveling: patients, families, elderly residents, and the staff and volunteers who meet them, all are drawn into a journey of the spirit," she said in a speech in 1981. Today, St Christopher's includes an in-patient facility as well as a program for at-home care. It provides interdisciplinary care led by nurses and all kinds of therapy services for living comfortably until death. Saunders often said, "You matter because you are you, and you matter to the last moment of your life. We will do all that we can not only to help you die peacefully, but also to live until you die."

That is a nursing perspective—after all, nursing was the career Saunders chose before other considerations intervened. Hospice lends itself to being nurse-led because it is a kind of care that is not focused on a cure but on close attention to each patient and their family and to their overall comfort. But Saunders also conceived of hospice as a truly interdisciplinary form of care that relied on input from physicians, social workers, clergy, and volunteers from the community. At the time, everything about this practice was radical: It was not strictly hierarchical. It included women in caring professions as experts and leaders. It centered on the patient and their family. And it held that patients should be in control of their own care.

This hospice model came to the United States when, in 1963, Florence Wald, RN (no relation to Lillian Wald), then the dean of the

Yale School of Nursing, became fascinated with Saunders's ideas and invited her to give a series of lectures. Wald was absolutely lit up by Saunders. "She made an indelible impression on me, for until then I had thought nurses were the only people troubled by how a terminal illness was treated," she writes. (A statement that is somewhat ironic given that Saunders *was* a nurse as well as a physician.) Wald stepped down from Yale to form an interdisciplinary team, and in 1974, that team founded the first modern hospice in the United States: Connecticut Hospice, in Branford, which to this day provides both home and inpatient/residential care. In 1978, Linda Kilburn, a social worker, founded Good Shepherd, the first hospice organization in Massachusetts, which also provides both home and residential care. When they were launched, these kinds of organizations were rare and operated on the margins, rooted in community, run by scrappy, visionary people who were deeply committed to the ideals Saunders articulated.

In 1983, hospice expanded when it was established as a Medicare benefit, a set plan of covered care for those with an estimated six months or less to live. Medicare pays a flat daily fee per patient to hospice organizations, which is meant to average out to cover all the costs for the terminal illness. The fact that hospice patients must generally forgo curative care certainly doesn't mean they go without medical care: medical care that is aimed toward comfort and well-being is the focus, and curative treatment for any disease not related to the terminal illness can be continued as usual. The Medicare benefit enabled hospice to be rolled out all over the country, and more people could access it. The percentage of people who choose to die in hospice has roughly doubled since then. But as the care model gets scaled up and becomes more profit-driven, it runs the risk of leaving its values behind.

Good Shepherd is engaged in the tricky balancing act of working within this financial system while maintaining its original radical values. The organization is notable in a few ways: First, its CEO, Timothy Boon, BS, RN, prioritizes the patient-nurse relationship and understands the variability inherent in each nurse-patient visit. Second, as several nurses on staff told me, nurses there usually have the time and resources to provide the best care they can—and that is rare.

Boon said that Good Shepherd's financial margins are very thin, partly because its leaders are careful to limit nurse caseloads as much as possible—and that's expensive, but it's also the foundation of hospice. Boon refuses to have nurses take on more patients than they can properly care for. Usually, he said, Good Shepherd's limit is about ten patients per nurse, with an eye toward mixing acuity, so that one nurse doesn't have ten patients all in need of intense management at the same time. Ideally, this makes for a very busy but not impossible schedule. At other hospices, especially for-profit ones, Boon said, it is not uncommon for one nurse to have to cover fifteen to twenty patients.

Boon explained that hospice works best, both for patients and for a hospice's finances, if people enter hospice when they still have at least a couple of months to live. When patients enter with just a few days or a week left, it's hard for them to benefit fully from the program. And for hospice organizations, that flat daily fee works best if a patient is enrolled for a certain span of time between admission (which is expensive) and death (which is expensive). This relatively uneventful span of time—when patients can benefit from improved pain control, spiritual care, music therapy, and the like—is rewarding for everyone, and the daily flat fee average allows the hospice to continue operating, albeit with narrow profit margins.

But narrow profit margins and a focus on therapeutic relationships aren't necessarily appealing to the more than 50 percent of hospice facilities in the United States that are now for profit. End-of-life care has become increasingly commercialized. In 2020, Rodney Mesquias, the owner of a chain of for-profit hospices in Texas, was sentenced to twenty years in prison for fraud and money laundering. He had aggressively recruited people in long-term care and group homes who were suffering from dementia and Alzheimer's, falsely telling them that they had only six months to live and even sending unsuspecting chaplains to discuss last rites. Mesquias enrolled these patients in unnecessary hospice services, which prevented them from accessing other, needed treatments. He kept patients, some with diminished mental capacity, on his hospice rolls for years, collecting $150 million from Medicare, which he used to buy luxury cars, jewelry, season sports tickets, and real estate and to ply physicians with parties and bottle service at Las Vegas nightclubs.

Meanwhile, Good Shepherd is about as close to Saunders's original vision of hospice care as one can find in the United States. It employs sixty-six direct-care nurses, eighteen social workers, three spiritual care providers, two physicians, and two music therapists. These providers are divided into roughly three teams, and each team holds weekly meetings to report updates on each patient, share ideas, and ask questions. I sat in on one of these meetings, which lasted about two hours.

Each update had the texture of real life, with attention paid to the details of each patient.

> "She woke up agitated, trying to take off her nightgown, family gave lorazepam.... She is that kind of strong spirit."

> "She doesn't want to keep holding on."

> "She appears to have lost weight and is increasingly confused. Jeff offered music and held her hand.... Her aide fixes her hair beautifully with a bun on top."

"The family is coming together, laughing over funny stories
and sharing photos. They were trying to place him in a
nursing home, but now feel it was better that he died at
home."

"Diagnosed with Alzheimer's fifteen years ago . . . He's been
married sixty years, they met as teenagers . . . Patient is a
psychologist. He and his wife loved to travel and have one
daughter . . . Family described him as a kind gentle person.
Devastating to see the impact of this disease on him."

When my mother died from breast cancer, her care was nothing
like this; it was more like a gauntlet we traveled together as I scram-
bled unsuccessfully to help the providers see her as a person, my most
beloved person. Toward the end, she was hospitalized at a small community hospital with what must have been the end stages of meta-
static cancer, but her oncologist was an hour away, in Boston, and
no one seemed to be able to say for sure what was happening. Six
weeks before her death, she was placed on a ventilator because of respiratory distress and then taken off it ten days later, able to breathe
on her own. I struggled to get one doctor to speak to another until,
finally, her oncologist in Boston called to deputize me to explain to
my mother that her cancer had spread to her liver and lungs and that
she was dying. He could not come to the community hospital, and he
didn't call a local physician who might have been able to deliver this
news. A social worker saw me crying in the hall. I told her I had to tell
my mother that her cancer had spread and she was dying. The social
worker said no—I should not be the one to tell my mother she was
dying, that I needed to get a medical professional to tell her, that this
was my mother's right. But which one? I didn't know—no one seemed
to know. A few days ticked by, and it turned out that was all we had.

This was how my mother came to die in a rehabilitation center attached to a hospital without being informed that her condition had changed and that she was dying—without being able to say goodbye, without hospice measures or any choices at all. In those very last days, the only medical professional who came to our aid in any meaningful way was the nurse who explained that my mother's ragged, gasping breath was a normal part of dying and that I didn't need to be afraid; that I should sit with her. By then, she was unconscious, and she didn't come back.

For so long, I told this story to myself in a way that was partly true: that my mother absolutely did not want to admit that death was coming; she wanted, so badly, to live. She had survived with cancer for fifteen years. She had to find a way to coexist with it, and her way was to simply ignore the likelihood that she would die, to just keep going. And, for a long time, this worked for her. I think she found ease in not asking too many questions. Second-guessing the physicians was not how she wanted to spend her finite time and energy.

Now I think about it a little differently: She deserved to have someone else take some responsibility for what was happening. Someone should have had the strength to wrestle the truth into that room, once it became clear. But things had not changed that much since Cicely Saunders sat with David Tasma. It was just easier for the physicians to suggest one more treatment, to elide my mother's prognosis when she didn't push to hear it. Without exactly lying, they acted as if they had a fix. And when it was finally obvious they didn't, they essentially disappeared. They just let her go.

Hospice is still radical. My mother's experience was surely more common than, for instance, Ahmad's experience. The practices on which hospice is based are not as valued in American health care as they should be. After all, when done ethically, hospice is not very profitable. It is not hierarchical. It is not completely quantifiable. There will never be the discovery of a cure for death.

One of nursing's greatest and most unique strengths is working within those electric moments of transition, in not pretending to have all the answers, not insisting on being in charge. When the potential for cure disappears, nurses are still there, still nursing. There's always something more to be done.

This was never clearer than at Ward 5B at San Francisco General Hospital. A nurse-led AIDS ward, 5B was a de facto hospice at a time when there was no treatment for this acquired immune deficiency syndrome and when those with the disease died within weeks or months. The ward was born out of one nurse's realization that AIDS patients needed end-of-life care they weren't getting, mainly because of the homophobic stigma and panic around AIDS at the time.

"I saw patients alone, begging for someone to come assist them," says Cliff Morrison, MSM, ACRN, in the 2018 documentary 5B. He recalls how AIDS patients in hospitals were basically abandoned, left without even food or clean sheets, a problem that only worsened as the virus and the panic spread. So, in 1983, Morrison volunteered to create a ward specifically for AIDS patients. Twelve other nurses, galvanized by what they had seen, joined him. They were worried about being infected themselves, but more than that, they were angry about how these patients were being treated. "How could you not provide the care that you knew how to do?" Alison Moed, RN, asked.

The ward filled quickly—with young people, many in their twenties, who were dying painful and frightening deaths, often after seeing friends die in the same way. Sometimes they were estranged from their families and felt very alone. The nurses tending to them deployed every kind of palliative care imaginable: Anyone could come visit. Sometimes a pet could be smuggled in, too. The nurses held brunch parties every weekend, at which a local performer wearing bunny ears served cake and other treats to those who could still enjoy them. And, crucially, the nurses provided human touch: hands-on nursing care. This was not happening anywhere else—elsewhere, AIDS patients were dying amid providers who were terrified of them. "If we can't save these folks, we are going to touch them," Morrison says in the documentary.

By the time Morrison created his AIDS ward, it was swiftly becoming an educated guess that whatever caused AIDS was not spread by casual contact—and, in fact, the human immunodeficiency virus, or HIV, would be identified that same year. So, the nurses sat up with the patients who had night sweats, changing their sheets as many times as necessary. "This was a tangible thing you could do. Wash them, put moisturizer on them," Mary Magee, RN, remembers. One patient who appears in the documentary, lying in his bed, emaciated, his eyes huge, says, "I had no human contact for a year. You forget love. When someone does touch you . . ." He closes his eyes. "Wow."

The nurses of 5B were soothing as much of that "total pain" as possible. As Magee says in the film, "You were allowed to love your patients." Of course, every single bit of this was controversial at the time, and the pushback was swift and furious: Some nurses and physicians found the premise of the ward offensive; the nursing union got involved. But the nurses of 5B kept going, through legal challenges and harassment, and they did not stop providing that care until the world had changed and the ward was closed in 2003.

It was no accident that 5B was a nurse-led ward. Good Shepherd hospice nurse Jerry Soucy, CHPN, RN argues that hospice is inherently nursing care. He told me about a time a physician on Twitter asked for suggestions about how physicians could lead difficult end-of-life conversations. Soucy said he objected to the framing of the question: "Don't let this be led by physicians. Not only are physicians *the worst* at it—categorically and almost universally—but also, it's really not appropriate to their role as physicians. They *see* it as their role because they see *everything* as their role. But it's really not an appropriate use of their discipline. Should physicians participate? Yes. Lead? No."

Forty-five years ago, when Soucy was a freshly graduated, twenty-one-year-old nurse at Augusta General Hospital in Maine (now MaineGeneral Health), he had an encounter that changed the way he thought about nursing. He was working in the intensive care unit when a man was brought in directly from the operating room. The surgeon had repaired an aneurysm in the patient's abdominal aorta, the largest artery in the body, which descends from the heart through the center of the torso, supplying blood to major organs. As Soucy remembered it, the scene was chaotic as the man, with organ damage and a huge new incision, was wheeled into the ICU while being hand-bagged for respiration. Three nurses, a respiratory therapist, the anesthesiologist, and a surgeon were starting multiple IVs, calling out directions, entering settings into the ventilator, connecting the man to the ventilator, sliding him onto the bed. And then the man started to wake up: his anesthesia was wearing off. "They were putting him on the vent, and he was bucking the vent, right? He's choking. The alarms are going off," Soucy told me.

Soucy got down next to the man's head and put his mouth next to his ear. He used what he called his FM radio announcer's voice. "I just said, 'Hey, this is where you are. This is what's going on. You're okay. We're going to take care of you.' And the guy chilled." As he told me this, all these decades later, Soucy's voice cracked. He said this was a formative moment for him. I asked him why. "I certainly got a sense of his panic," he said. "I looked at the other people, focusing on their tasks, which obviously needed to be done. But I also had this feeling of 'Hey, what are we doing? Wait a minute. Stop making all this noise.

Stop with the hustle. Do we need these three other people in here? What matters most? What does this guy *need*?'"

Soucy knew that the patient needed the medical interventions he was getting—and he did survive—but that was not *all* he needed. Soucy thinks of his nursing practice as providing intelligent care based on the answers to these questions: What does this person want? What does this person need? What matters the most right now? These three questions inform all he does in hospice.

Soucy described a recent hospice patient visit: The elderly woman was dying from congestive heart failure and kidney failure, at home, surrounded by loved ones. But she had had a difficult night with agitated delirium, a common effect of the body's slowly shutting down, and one family member had tried to help by talking to her loudly and even holding her down, which only made things worse. Soucy's colleague, the nurse on call, arrived at 3 a.m., took stock of the dying woman's agitation and of the exhausted family members, and decided that what mattered most right then was sleep. So, he gave the dying woman a sedative, and everyone slept. When Soucy walked in the next day, one family member was quietly holding the dying woman's hand. The woman's breath was gurgling, the common symptom of approaching death.

Soucy wanted to keep everyone calm. He slipped behind the recliner where the dying woman lay and put his hands on her reassuringly. The family member holding the dying woman's hand said she was a massage therapist and asked if she should rub the woman's feet. Soucy, a big smile breaking behind his white beard, said, "Oh yeah!" Then, from behind the recliner, he asked someone to get an oral syringe of the hydromorphone to help ease the woman's breathing discomfort. He talked to the woman soothingly, walking her through what was happening: "You're home. People are here." He modeled calm for the family. He thinks of caring for a dying person as being like landing a plane: very gradual adjustments, nothing sudden, a slow and gradual descent, a gentle touchdown. A trust fall.

Sandarovscaia also feels that attentive nursing can make a gentle death possible. One of her patients, with pancreatic cancer, had painful fluid build-up in her abdomen. She went to the hospital to have five liters drained, but then the fluid built up again. The woman did not want to go back to get it drained again, but she confided in Sandarovscaia that she was afraid of disappointing her family, afraid they would think she didn't want to fight for more days of life. Sandarovscaia helped the woman gather her children and her husband, so that she could explain this to them: She was tired, and she wanted to stop. Her family understood.

Sandarovscaia thought about what a difference it made to let the truth into the room. "And she died very peacefully. They all gathered together. She took her last breath with everyone there." They held her as she fell; they didn't let her go.

CHAPTER 6

AUTONOMY

The Fight for Choices: A Complicated Story of Nurses, Birth Control, and Abortion

In February 1935, two young women walked into nurse Adele Gordon's birth control clinic in the bustling Plankinton Arcade building in downtown Milwaukee. One said she was married to a medical student; she and her husband already had an eighteen-month-old and could not afford another baby. The other said she was unmarried but wanted a birth control device. Gordon, following the law at the time, told the unmarried woman she could not help her. She then brought the married woman into her exam room, where she took a medical history, fitted her for a diaphragm, and gave her information on how to use it. She charged her five dollars. Before the women left, Gordon let them know that she would be holding a free lecture on birth control later that month.

About two weeks later, the married woman showed up at the clinic again, but this time she was with two police officers and Walter Drews, state Board of Health investigator. Drews had been to the clinic before. After receiving complaints from several church groups and one nursing organization, he'd come by incognito and asked to see the physician on site; there wasn't one. Gordon was an experienced nurse who had been providing birth control for many years. Her husband, John, helped her run the business. This time, Drews and the police officers seized all the materials at the clinic and hauled both Adele and John Gordon away in a squad car. It was illegal for nurses to provide birth control. Only a physician or pharmacist could do that.

Gordon had broken the law, and she must have fully expected to be convicted and sentenced to six months in prison. But after both she and John each posted $750 bail (about $16,000 today), she went on the offensive. As historian Rose Holz, PhD, has written, Gordon put up flyers all over town that read *Birth Control Is at Stake in the State of Wisconsin* and urged community members to fight to keep her clinic open. She and her supporters wrote to newspapers, labor leaders, and the ACLU, and Gordon wrote to Margaret Sanger, a fellow nurse and prominent birth control advocate. Sanger wrote back with support and indignation on Gordon's behalf, though she herself had, by that time, already conceded birth control to (overwhelmingly male) physicians.

Gordon concocted a defense: She wasn't selling birth control; that was illegal. She was selling nursing services and information but giving away the diaphragms for free. Meanwhile, the fervor over the couple's arrest had Milwaukee rapt. On March 6, Gordon's resolute face was plastered on page 4 of the *Milwaukee Sentinel Extra* under the headline "Posts Bond." The jury selection was contentious because so many on the panel held strong religious views against birth control and had to be dismissed. Finally, the six members of the jury were chosen, five men and one woman.

The courtroom was packed for Adele Gordon's trial. The *Milwaukee Journal* set the scene: "Gray haired women of grandmother age, matrons in their forties, men far beyond the age of innocence and boys seemingly still of high school age and young girls crammed the courtroom." When Gordon took the stand, she seems to have decided to make the most of the situation by educating the crowd, to such an extent that the judge had to ask her to stop turning the trial into a lecture on birth control. Constantly interrupted by objections, Gordon steadfastly argued that contraception was a boon for all people. She said that her pamphlets were not indecent but instructive. Yes, she had supplied birth control, but for free, she argued, and she had provided it within the standard practices of the worldwide birth control movement. Furthermore, she went on, she was fully qualified as a nurse to do so. She detailed her earlier work as a visiting nurse, when she saw the consequences of involuntary motherhood repeatedly: "I became interested in birth control work as I entered the homes of the poor and saw women overburdened with children—"

At this, the assistant district attorney jumped up, shouting his objection. "That is hearsay and highly prejudicial, what she saw in the poor to arouse her interest in birth control." But none of this was a secret; in fact, some women in the courthouse openly wept to hear about a problem that was intimately familiar. It was obvious that women had more pregnancies than they wanted or, sometimes, could survive—what was less obvious was exactly how to prevent them. The crowd in the courtroom was treated to more expert information about birth control that March day in 1935 than many of them could legally have gotten anywhere else.

The jury deliberated for just twenty-five minutes before finding Gordon not guilty. About two weeks later, her husband, John, was also acquitted. The very next month, an advertisement appeared in the *Milwaukee Journal* advertising the Gordons' free birth control lectures and clinic, open once more. Of course, technically, the Gordons had been guilty, but a change in public opinion was gathering force—birth control would not be a crime forever. Nurses were instrumental in turning that tide. But the story of nurses and midwives, birth control and abortion, is a complicated one.

From one perspective, nurses and midwives across all times and places have been some of the fiercest advocates and most essential providers of reproductive care. Michelle Drew, DNP, CNM, who is descended from midwives going back at least ten generations, explains that traditional midwives routinely provided full-spectrum care: people who gave birth one month might have needed advice on how to use a sponge for contraception the next month, or an abortifacient tea the following year. This is consistent with nursing as a holistic discipline.

But there's a tendency in modern professional nursing to seek respectability, to uphold hierarchies, and to avoid controversy. Nursing organizations and schools have often shied away from teaching and supporting reproductive care as an integral part of nursing practice. Some nurses and midwives argue that this is unethical and antithetical to nursing. After all, people need full-spectrum reproductive care, and nurses have a unique role in providing it.

This push-pull was embodied by Margaret Sanger, a nurse and the founder of Planned Parenthood, who advanced access to modern birth control. But in seeking political respectability for her cause, Sanger supported eugenics, the racist, ableist, and anti-Semitic population pseudoscience that argued that only certain "fit" people should have children. Sanger's prototypical (and illegal) birth control clinic, which she opened in Brooklyn in 1916, is one way we have arrived at this moment when effective birth control is—for the time being, at least—an established part of a right to privacy, whereas before it had been variously inaccessible, ineffective, and illegal. But it is equally true that the reprehensible compromises Sanger struck for the sake of political acceptance have also led us to today, when reproductive care is being curtailed and threatened.

Contraception and abortion have been used all over the world from antiquity onward, and they have always been part of midwifery and community nursing care, whether legal or illegal. Though cultural attitudes toward pregnancy and family planning have differed, the actual methods were much the same. Practices such as withdrawal or barriers over the penis were often used, though they were complicated by human nature or the fact that they relied on men to cooperate. Women used vaginal suppositories, sponges, or douches; they chewed roots or brewed herbal teas to prevent or end pregnancy. Enslaved women in the United States, for instance, chewed cotton root as a contraceptive or abortifacient. Indigenous Mexican women chewed the root of a wild yam, which was later used in the development of the birth control pill. Remedy books from the European Middle Ages often contain herb concoctions to bring about a missed period, which was often understood as a way either to boost fertility or to induce abortion. These old methods often had a high rate of failure and complications, but they were not necessarily ineffective. None of this is to suggest that the pre-twentieth century was a time of effective family planning—it was mostly the opposite—but all kinds of sexual and reproductive care were historically part of skilled midwives' and nurses' practice, and people ably used what was available.

Birth control and abortion were not always fraught political topics. In the early United States through the mid-1800s, both birth control and abortion were legal. (Though enslaved Black women were always prohibited from both.) In the 1850s, for instance, about one in every five or six pregnancies ended in abortion. But then the political atmosphere took a turn, and by the 1880s, all states had laws restricting abortion. And birth control became criminalized with the

Comstock Laws of 1873, which categorized contraception as obscene and outlawed the distribution of information about it.

None of these laws meant contraception and abortion weren't being used or weren't necessary. Nurses and midwives had special insight into exactly how necessary they were. After all, it is one thing to know in theory what happens when a woman gets pregnant over and over again, but quite another to be the one called to the aftermath of an unsafe abortion or to try to keep a woman alive through her eleventh birth in as many years.

Margaret Sanger had two formative experiences: One was watching her devout Irish-Catholic mother die of tuberculosis at the age of fifty after being relentlessly worn away by eleven births and seven miscarriages. Sanger remembered her mother's life as one of unending drudgery: cooking, cleaning, bearing children, and caring for them. There was never enough money, food, or time to spare. Sanger had wanted to be a physician so she could help her mother, and she always believed that if she had had more medical knowledge, she might have saved her.

Then, in 1910, newly married and graduated from nursing school, Sanger moved to New York City and began working part time as a visiting nurse at the Henry Street Settlement, with Lillian Wald. The grinding poverty and back-to-back pregnancies she saw there would have reminded her of her own mother's life and early death. In her autobiography, Sanger wrote about how it felt to nurse these women, to be so intimately acquainted with their bodies: "These were not merely 'unfortunate conditions among the poor' such as we read about. I knew the women personally. They were living, breathing human beings, with hopes, fears and aspirations like my own, yet their weary, misshapen bodies . . . were destined to be thrown on the scrap heap before they were thirty-five. I could not escape from the facts of their wretchedness; neither was I able to see any way out."

On the Lower East Side around this time, about one-third of women knew of no birth control method at all aside from abortion, which was illegal. In her work, Sanger saw the many ways women attempted to induce abortion: herbs, turpentine, throwing themselves down flights of stairs, inserting knitting needles and hooks. Women would ask pharmacists and midwives for advice; some were helpful, but many were fearful of the law or ignorant of the methods themselves. Sanger wrote in her autobiography that she knew of "only two methods" to prevent pregnancy. She didn't specify what they were, except to say that they placed the responsibility on the husband, which was a problem. She wrote that she experienced her nursing as a kind of recurring nightmare in which pregnant women were carried off to the hospital and never came back, children were sent to institutions, women were found with their heads in the oven.

In the decades after, Sanger would always come back to the story of one woman who, she said, inspired her awakening. Sadie Sachs, a Russian-Jewish immigrant with three small children, had become septic after an abortion. Sanger nursed Sachs back to health in the family's tenement apartment. Sachs then begged a physician to tell her how to prevent pregnancy, saying, "Another baby will finish me." The physician told Sachs that she couldn't have her cake and eat it, too, and suggested she make her husband sleep on the roof. Sanger was called back to the apartment a few months later to find the husband distraught and Sachs unconscious from another abortion; this time, she died.

"I knew I could no longer go back to merely keeping people alive," Sanger writes. "I was finished with palliatives and superficial cures; I was resolved to . . . do something to change the destiny of mothers whose miseries were as vast as the sky." She wanted to find reliable ways to prevent pregnancies in the first place. Because Sanger was the founder of Planned Parenthood, many assume she was pro-abortion, but she opposed it, mainly because her understanding of abortion was shaped by what she saw in her nursing work: it was a risky procedure forced into the literal and figurative back alley. She had certainly not been trained in nursing school on how to perform a safe abortion—or provide birth control, for that matter.

The push to criminalize abortion in the first place was the work of the newly formed American Medical Association. Physicians, particularly within the new specialty of obstetrics and gynecology, were attempting to wrest control of reproductive care from midwives, who were often the ones providing abortions. The physicians' group demonized abortions in order to demonize midwifery care.

As ever, the effort to paint midwives and independent nurses as incompetent hags was not solely a matter of gender but also had overlays of race, class, and immigration bias. It was a matter of power and control, *and* it was a matter of business competition. Physicians leveled blame especially at Black and immigrant midwives, whom they portrayed as superstitious, dangerous foreign women—shades of witches. (In reality, some physicians provided abortions, as did other practitioners.)

The larger context was that birth rates were declining among U.S.-born white women; meanwhile, slavery ended, and immigration increased. There was concern about maintaining white Christian control of the country. In 1903, President Theodore Roosevelt was speaking to white women when he said "willful sterility" was an unforgivable sin. George Kosmak, a prominent gynecologist, was referring to women like Sadie Sachs when he wrote that it was necessary for the economy to have an underclass of workers who, as he put it, were characterized by quantity, not quality. At the same time, an official, federally funded program of forced sterilization targeted nonwhite and disabled people throughout the twentieth century.

These efforts were all connected—the movement to suppress

traditional nurse and midwifery practices, to put control in the hands of physicians, to sterilize marginalized people, and to prevent everyone else from obtaining birth control or abortion. It was a campaign to control the future of the country by controlling who provided reproductive care and who had babies.

Sanger became resolved to help women control their fertility *because* she was a nurse: She saw the problem in a visceral way through her patients. But because she had not been trained in reproductive care, first, she had to figure out how contraception actually worked. She read medical texts, and she went to France, where women had been passing down recipes and devices for contraception for generations. At the time, the best option was a diaphragm or pessary inserted into the vagina to cover the cervix, used with spermicide. So Sanger started spreading this information far and wide via pamphlets, even though this was illegal under the federal Comstock Laws, which were joined by various state laws that prohibited it further. In Connecticut, for instance, even the private *use* of contraception was illegal.

At the time, Sanger was heavily influenced by leftist politics and found that socialist labor organizers were more useful allies in distributing her pamphlets than the new feminists, who told her to wait until women had the vote to act on birth control. In particular, she was influenced by her mentor and fellow nurse Emma Goldman, who is better remembered as a labor activist and anarchist but who saw birth control as part of the larger rights of workers to control the circumstances of their lives.

Goldman had become a nurse when she was sent to prison on charges of inciting a riot for telling an audience that the poor had a sacred right to bread. While locked up, she became ill and was cared for at the hospital in the jail complex. After she recovered, a physician asked her to stay on as a nurse; he trained her and put her in charge of the sixteen-bed women's ward. She loved the work.

For the next decade, Goldman worked off and on as a nurse, and what she saw gave her total conviction in the necessity of birth control. She wrote that after nursing a woman through labor and delivery, "I would return home sick and distressed, hating the men responsible for the frightful condition of their wives and children, hating myself most of all because I did not know how to help them." She was often begged to perform abortions, but she always refused, believing them too dangerous, and she wrote that she didn't have good information on contraception to share with her patients—that is, until she started working with Sanger to distribute leaflets and magazines on birth control. As a result, she was arrested for violating the Comstock Laws at least twice.

Later, the two women became estranged as Goldman moved further into broader political radicalism and Sanger shifted away from radicalism and became a one-issue activist. But Sanger and Goldman are both, in their own ways, potent examples of the ways in which intellectual and political convictions are formed by nursing work and how, in turn, nursing work provides a concrete way to act on those convictions.

On October 16, 1916, Sanger took the next logical step: She opened a birth control clinic in Brownsville, Brooklyn, then a neighborhood of recent immigrants. In Yiddish, Italian, and English, she advertised the clinic's services as being an alternative to abortion for mothers who did not want or could not afford more children. At the clinic, Sanger and her sister Ethel Byrne, also a nurse, offered sex education and contraceptive advice. They recommended a particular pessary to prevent pregnancy. They did not fit women for the devices, but they explained how they worked—women who had had two children or more needed the larger size—and where to get them. (Pharmacies carried them because they were also used to prevent uterine prolapse.) A little more than a week after they'd opened the clinic, a Mrs.

Whitehurst came in to get a sex education pamphlet. The next day, she came back with police, who arrested Sanger and impounded all the clinic's supplies and furniture. Sanger was apoplectic. In the ten days the clinic was open, it had served 464 women.

Sanger was found guilty and sentenced to thirty days in a work-house. Her lawyers appealed the conviction, and a New York appeals court upheld the ruling but added an opinion that physicians could legally prescribe birth control for just about any medical reason, which had previously been illegal. This compromise was an inflection point. In 1921, Sanger opened another New York City clinic, but this time, one staffed by physicians. In complying with the physician-only mandate, she helped put the control of women's fertility back in the hands of a group that had done much to damage both the bodily autonomy of women and, not at all coincidentally, the independent practice of nurses and midwives.

Sanger never wavered in her dedication to birth control but became willing to ally herself with just about anyone in this quest. She famously spoke to the women of the Ku Klux Klan about contraception. She approved of the nonconsensual sterilization of the mentally "unfit" and thus harnessed the birth control movement to eugenic ideas. She ceded birth control to physicians, part of a shift in the idea of birth control as being a tool of liberation to one of population control. The fact that she did this *as a nurse* lent precious credibility to vicious and violent ideas.

In some ways, it worked: Sanger's tactics made the idea of birth control more palatable to those in power, and birth control slowly became more accepted. But those tactics meant it was not a victory for *everyone*, and not a durable victory—if control over one's own fertility must be granted, it can just as easily be taken away.

One lasting ramification of Sanger's willingness to make common cause with racists is that it has made it easy for reproductive care opponents to argue that birth control and abortion are a kind of genocide forced upon Black communities. Actually, Black communities had always used traditional methods of birth control and were perfectly capable of distinguishing between the movement to make reproductive care accessible and the racist ideas that some advocates of birth control held. Sanger worked closely with W. E. B. Du Bois, a birth control proponent, to set up clinics in Black neighborhoods. But it certainly wasn't just her: The birth control movement in Black communities had its own momentum and its own leaders. Notably, the National Association of Colored Graduate Nurses, directed by Mabel Staupers, RN—the very woman who broke down army nurse segregation in World War II—led the way in distributing birth control information and partnered with Negro Home Demonstration Clubs to reach people in rural areas.

Finally, in 1965, the U.S. Supreme Court ruled that married couples have a right to privacy that includes contraception. In 1973, *Roe v. Wade* established that pregnant women also have a privacy-based right to end a pregnancy, to a point. The latter ruling stood for nearly fifty years, but the original decision in *Roe* was not about abortion as a human right. It was instead predicated on a physician's autonomy. In the opinion, Justice Blackmun wrote, "The attending physician, in consultation with his patient, is free to determine, without regulation by the State, that, in his medical judgment, the patient's pregnancy should be terminated."

Sanger has been rightfully disavowed by Planned Parenthood, and scholars have discussed the ramifications of her embrace of eugenics. But her story illuminates something important about nursing and how it can work in the world. Nursing can be, and has been, a powerful force for human rights. But it is equally true that nursing can be, and has been, a powerful force *against* human rights. Sanger's story moves from one pole to the other, and can help us understand how we got here, to the current reproductive care landscape, for better and for worse.

With *Roe* now overturned, abortion criminalized in some states, and other privacy-based rights in jeopardy, reproductive care in the United States is more threatened than usual. And nurses and midwives are, again and always, stepping into that breach.

Michelle Drew's midwifery practice is both a response to what she sees as necessary in this moment and also a part of a long and unbroken tradition of Black midwifery that has always provided reproductive care, including birth control and abortion. "Every generation of my family going back to 1750, there's been a midwife," Drew said.

Her practice, the Ubuntu Black Family Wellness Collective, in Wilmington, Delaware, is a free clinic in the service of reproductive justice: Any community member can walk in at any time, no appointment necessary, and walk out with the birth control of their choice. Or they can get pills for a medication abortion. Or they can get prenatal and obstetrics care—choosing to give birth with Drew at home or in the nearby hospital. They can bring their mother, their children, their partner. They can get doula care, breastfeeding support, and nutrition advice. They can get acupressure and reflexology and Drew's special ginger or peppermint tinctures for nausea, made from recipes passed down from her grandmother. In fact, Ubuntu is a living tribute to the expert community midwifery practiced by Drew's grandmother. It is almost a portal to a different world, one where this kind of care was never suppressed. Ubuntu is Drew's reimagining of what is possible, an answer to the medical system's failure to safely care for pregnant Black people. As such, it is innovative and radical—but also nothing new.

Drew spent her summers with her grandparents and cousins in the family's small Virginia town. Every day, her grandmother went out for home visits, but everyone in the community knew that if her front door was open, they could just come by. If she was cooking dinner, she'd lower the burner flame, set one of her grandchildren in front of the pot to watch it, and send the other grandchildren outside to play. Then she'd direct her attention to how she could care for her neighbor. She never made people feel like her time was more valuable than theirs.

Drew was awed by the respect her grandmother commanded. "It was like walking around town with a celebrity, almost someone who had a semi-divine status, because she cared for so many people." Her grandmother's practice was intensely tactile: She hugged and touched people easily. She could cure a child's stomachache or fever with a concoction made in her kitchen. Drew didn't take Tylenol until she was an adult.

Drew saw her first birth at age three, when her grandmother went to help a woman in labor and brought her along. She stayed out of the way and watched her grandmother moving deliberately to comfort and support the birthing woman. Her grandmother was quiet and patient, seeming to know what to do out of intrinsic knowledge—what Drew and other Black midwives call mother wit—and deep confidence. Even as a three-year-old, Drew felt the magnetism of her grandmother's work.

At Ubuntu, Drew brings the traditional midwifery her foremothers practiced to her own community. Her open-door policy is a re-creation of her grandmother's welcoming front door, and the care she provides comes from different ways of knowing: the ancient, tactile mother wit, herbalist knowledge she learned from her grandmother; and the pharmacology and physiology knowledge from her doctorate of nursing and nurse-midwifery training. When a client has morning sickness, Drew makes them herbal tinctures before she prescribes pharmaceuticals. If a patient has a bladder infection, she prescribes antibiotics and talks to them about ways to increase the acidity of their urine, to make a repeat infection less likely. She knows which pressure points in the body bring on labor, ease pain. She almost never does cervical exams while a person is in labor—instead she feels her patients' legs for what she describes as a creeping coldness that moves from the feet upward as the cervix opens. A lot of her practice involves making people feel loved and valued. "To have a healthy pregnancy, most of us need to be well fed, well supported, well loved and well rested," she said.

Drew has another early memory, and it is not a good one: Her great-grandmother and grandmother had been summoned to the local health department, and Drew went with them. There, a white physician and nurse told her grannies that their midwife permits were no longer valid. Now that there were roads and hospitals and obstetricians, the two women were no longer needed, they were told. As Drew recounted this, she swallowed back tears.

The roots of that moment, the taking of their permits, lay in the Sheppard-Towner Act of 1921, also known as the National Maternity and Infancy Protection Act, which provided funding for infant and maternal health programs but also regulated midwives in a way that sought to sideline and then eradicate them—particularly Black midwives, who provided the vast majority of reproductive care in the South. The law was brutally effective: one hundred years later, only 6 percent of nurse midwives are Black. Despite such laws, Drew and others like her are still here.

It is within this sweeping historical context that Drew views the provision of abortion care, which is currently legal and protected in Delaware. She says she will find a way to make sure her patients are served, no matter what comes. Full-spectrum reproductive care, including abortion and contraception, is what midwives like her grandmother provided, and it is what she will continue to provide.

Prompted by the overturning of *Roe* and the long decades of restricted access that came first, other nurses are thinking outside mainstream boundaries, too. Medication abortion is one key tool nurses and midwives are using to maintain access to safe abortion, as clinics close or become harder to get to and abortion services go underground. Medication abortion (an alternative to surgical or procedural abortion) is the combination of mifepristone and miso-prostol, which, when taken at intervals, function to block progester-one, a pregnancy hormone, and cause contractions, safely inducing an abortion at up to twelve weeks' gestation. (It is also used to re-solve a miscarriage.) In eighteen states and Washington, DC, nurse practitioners can prescribe the drugs, though the other thirty-two states restrict their prescription to physicians, as a way of reducing access altogether. The development of this medication regimen has completely changed abortion care since it was last illegal in the early 1970s, when options were limited to procedures that could be dan-gerous outside a clinical setting. Access to a pill that can be taken at home is much harder to restrict than access to a surgical procedure. In fact, there are websites for groups that provide the pills by mail (particularly the Netherlands-based AidAccess), even facilitating ac-cess in U.S. states where it is illegal. The World Health Organization has reported that the two-drug combination is extremely safe and effective, and research suggests that it can be safely taken at home via a telemedicine consultation or, in some cases, in the absence of any clinical care at all.

Stephanie, MSN, CNM, is a certified nurse-midwife who was pre-viously with Planned Parenthood and now works for Hey Jane, a new telehealth provider of medication abortion. She came to midwifery through her work as a visiting nurse. On home visits, she developed close relationships with her patients and their families, who shared all kinds of personal stories and questions with her. "They'd say, 'My sister-in-law is pregnant, and she wants an abortion, and she's not sure, can I ask you questions about that? Does that affect your fertility later?' Or, 'I heard you can buy misoprostol on the street; is that true?' Those types of conversations," Stephanie recalled. "I get teary thinking about it. Because, yes, it is a recognition of the long history of midwives providing full-spectrum care to women in their communities. But, for me, it was even more than that. It was the opportunity to be in people's lives. And they trusted me."

These home visits led Stephanie to choose a midwifery school where she knew she would get training in abortion (which is rare), because no matter what her patients needed, she wanted to be able to offer it. She now provides a very different kind of care from what she provided before. "I felt like it was my personal responsibility to go back to working in abortion care, because this way, I can directly impact access," she said. "But this is the least patient-facing job I've ever had, in terms of how much time I actually spend with patients." Still, she pointed out that the nursing she provides now is *also* home care. It's just that she appears on a screen or in a text chat, not physically in the patient's living room. Sometimes, especially now, telehealth is the most patient-centered way to provide abortion care.

Many patients, Stephanie said, live in areas of the United States that are hostile to abortion, and they are afraid to go to a clinic. They might be on active duty in the military and not want anyone to know. They may not want to walk past protesters, or the only clinic might be hours away. They may not be able to get time off work. Some just prefer to be at home; they find it more comfortable.

It works like this: If you live in a state where Hey Jane is authorized to provide abortion pills, you can go to its website, where you'll answer a few questions about your last period, your health, and your birth control use. If a patient would like a face-to-face telehealth visit with a provider, she can have one, but it's not required, and Stephanie says the majority of patients don't want one. Often, it is safe for the patient to end her pregnancy with the pills. In this case, Stephanie will approve the medication, and it will be sent in the mail, along with detailed instructions and information on what to expect. For any concerns, a provider is on call twenty-four hours a day via text, phone, or teleconference. There is a flat fee of $249 for the whole process, and financial aid is available from abortion funds, nationwide grassroots organizations that help people afford abortions.

Even nurses who don't provide abortions themselves have an important role to play in helping patients find the care they need. But the legal landscape around abortion in the United States is shifting quickly, and nurses in states where abortion is restricted are often left wondering what they can do or say. Because there are no clear guidelines for nurses, nursing schools often avoid the subject entirely. Anna Brown, BSN, RN, director of education at Nurses for Sexual and Reproductive Health, tries to fill that gap. She runs classes and workshops to help nurses understand how to meet their ethical obligation to patients without jeopardizing their nursing licenses or putting themselves at legal risk. For instance, she teaches nurses about mandatory reporting laws. Some nurses think they are obligated to report patients they think may have self-managed their own abortion. Actually, Brown explains, there is no legal reason a nurse would ever need to report this, and in fact, nursing ethics does not allow it, as it does harm to the patient.

When nurses are unsure where the legal lines fall, they can be reluctant to take any action at all. Part of Brown's job is to delineate those lines for them, so they are more likely to help as much as they can. For instance, in places where abortion is illegal, nurses can't legally provide procedural abortion or abortion pills, but they can tell patients about their options for traveling out of state to get a legal abortion. They also can't give medical advice about self-managing an abortion. When this is the issue, Brown says, the nurses' role can be to educate very generally about the existence of abortion pills and how they work, without specifically counseling the patient. Nurses can state that both the World Health Organization and the U.S. Food and Drug Administration say that abortion pills are safe and effective. They can describe how some people get the pills and how some people use them.

"For a nurse, the line between giving medical advice and giving information is really removing the word *you*," Brown said. This sounds simple, but it can be difficult: "Nurses are used to connecting, and they're used to giving medical information. All of a sudden, you have to move to the third person [when speaking to a patient]. It's uncomfortable and odd, but that's the delineation. You would say, 'The way the abortion pills work is by inducing a miscarriage. If someone were to take those pills, they would be able to tell a health care professional that they think they're experiencing a miscarriage. Scientifically, there's no way to test for those medications in the blood or urine.'"

Brown points out that community leaders, both online and off, are important for connecting patients to sources for these pills, as nurses and other health care workers have to protect their licenses. "You could say something like 'Hey, I see that you're having a lot of questions. It sounds like you prefer to take these pills at home, but there's not a clinic in your area. There are websites that can offer you more support around this than I can.'"

Brown's work is especially necessary because, even for nurses who are interested in this work, it is not easy to find training, jobs, or even information. While nurses are routinely trained in labor and delivery, other kinds of care, like abortion and even birth control, are often seen as taboo or too stigmatized to teach, research, or practice.

Nurse scientist Monica McLemore, PhD, RN, is working to break down those barriers. She believes that nurses can be instrumental in creating a completely different world. In order to define both the problem and the solution, McLemore headed a study that described the barriers to nurses' providing abortion care and described strategies to increase nurse career pathways into abortion care. The study found that recruitment and retention strategies work, but that more concrete action is needed to improve these educational and professional pathways, so that nurses who want to work in reproductive health can find their way in and thrive there. The fact that so many nursing and midwifery schools don't train in abortion is certainly not helping.

McLemore's work is grounded in reproductive justice, a framework developed by Black women in the 1990s. Reproductive justice advocates for the rights of all people to freely choose to get pregnant or not, to stay pregnant or not, and to parent their children in a safe and healthy environment without interference. "I come from the tradition of Nurse-Family Partnership. I come from the tradition of [the] Centering Pregnancy [program] and group prenatal care," McLemore said in a talk in April 2022, citing nurse-led programs that have been shown to be transformative. She argued for the vast potential in the nursing workforce to respond to the need for reproductive care: "That was all started by public health nursing and midwives! We can unleash the creativity of our profession and our discipline again if that's where we decide we want to make our resources investment."

Nurses who work in abortion care echoed this in conversations—a frustrating clash between nursing's huge potential to address patients' need for abortion and nursing's reluctance to get visibly involved in abortion. All the nurses I spoke to who provide abortion care had to go out of their way to seek the training they needed and felt that nursing as a whole had a responsibility that it was failing to live up to.

One nurse practitioner, whom I'll call Hannah, provides abortion and works in the Washington, DC, area. "Truly, in most nursing programs, they are really not addressing contraception, much less abortion care. That is a significant problem," she says, detailing how difficult it is for nurses to get the necessary training and education. "It's tough to then speak of nursing as a whole and how we deal with this, because, as a *whole*, we don't."

Julie Jenkins, DNP, APRN, specializes in sexual and reproductive care as a provider, educator, and advocate. She puts it this way: "The only women's health training that people get in nursing programs is maternal and child health. It's not sexual reproductive health. It's not gender and reproductive health. None of those things. It's maternal and child health. Those are combined into one thing. And generally, no one ever mentions abortion."

When Jenkins was a doctoral student at the Johns Hopkins University School of Nursing, she bumped up against what she sees as nursing's very calculated avoidance of these topics. For her research, she proposed a quality improvement project that would look at how to train primary care nurse practitioners in medication abortions, but she was unable to get Johns Hopkins's institutional approval for the project as described. She says she was encouraged to do the project for the same drug combination, but *only* with regard to the drugs' use to resolve early miscarriage, not for abortion. She moved forward with this, only to be told again she could not get approval. This back-and-forth went on for a year. No one ever stated point-blank that she could not research medication abortions; they simply continued to stonewall her. Her adviser told her she'd never seen anything like it. "It's abortion stigma," Jenkins said. "Misoprostol and mifepristone have the safety profile of Tylenol. There's no reason. It's political." She believes that nursing is forever wedded to being inoffensive—

a gendered concern—and that topics like abortion challenge the very foundation of nursing.

But Jenkins refuses to give up. For her, pointing out nursing's failures is a way to claim and create a different vision of nursing. This insistence on reimagining a better world is nursing, too. Some nurses *are* finding innovative ways to provide reproductive care, ways that nimbly respond to our current realities and that echo the work of past nurses and midwives.

I asked Brown how she combatted feelings of hopelessness. She said, "Having a historical understanding of how professional nurses and midwives have always served our community is really helpful. Regardless of what is going on, the priority has always been the health and wellness of our community members." For all the complications inherent in the history of nursing and reproductive care, pull one thread and—as Brown points out—it can become clear, if not simple: What do people need and how can nurses provide it?

CHAPTER 7

ENVIRONMENT

Seeing the Future: Nursing in a Swiftly
Changing Climate

When the surge from Superstorm Sandy sluiced into Manhattan on a Monday night in 2012, twelve feet of floodwater poured into the basement of NYU Langone Health medical center. The entire electrical system for the building is located in the basement, and so, at around 7:45 that evening, the hospital blinked into darkness. The whir and hiss of ventilators and IV pumps ceased as the wind rattled the hospital windows. Almost immediately, the emergency generators on the roof brought the power back on, but the relief was short-lived. As the storm battered the city, the roof generators started to fail, too. One of the most advanced hospitals in the country, a 450-bed facility filled with patients dependent on every kind of medical technology, was dark and quiet.

In the NICU, tiny premature babies were on life support devices that included incubators and ventilators, and now there was no electricity to run them. The NICU nurses had never been in a situation like this before. Nevertheless, they sprang into action. They started with the sickest, most fragile babies, the ones who were dependent on the technology to stay alive, bundling them onto warming pads and covering them with blankets. They attached the babies' airway tubes to plastic bulbs, and the nurses squeezed the bulbs to deliver air directly to the babies' lungs, substituting for the ventilators. This is called hand-bagging, and it is painstaking: The total air capacity of the lungs of a two-pound baby is something like two tablespoons. If you squeeze too much air in, their lungs can rupture. Then, while still hand-bagging, a team of five carried each baby down nine flights of stairs in the dark, their steps illuminated only by flashlights.

That evening, the nurses successfully evacuated all the babies from the NICU, some of the most critically ill patients at the hospital and only some of the 215 patients evacuated that night. Bellevue Hospital, just down First Avenue from NYU Langone, evacuated 725. Most of the evacuations were carried out by nurses, in coordination with other staff, as mobile and landline phone service in the city cut in and out.

Most news outlets covered what happened that night as a feel-good hero story instead of the beginning of a worldwide horror movie, but it is just as much one as the other. Climate change–driven hurricanes, floods, heat waves, and wildfires are already impacting human health all over the world in ways big and small. Nurses are the first responders to these crises, and their roles in both responding to and mitigating the health impacts will only become more important as the effects of climate change multiply. Nurses are trained to think about the patient in the context of their environment, and they are adept at noticing patterns in people's health and developing plans to tackle them. Nursing climate change, like climate change itself, involves a spectrum of events, from evacuating babies one at a time in a crisis, to using school policy to mitigate increased asthma rates in children, to researching heat-related kidney failure in agricultural workers. Nurses are not always understood as crucial to climate change response, but they should be, because they *are* uniquely situated to respond.

We might think of climate change as a future problem, but it is here now and has been for decades. This is just some of what nurses are already noticing: With increased heat and decreased air quality comes increased risk of preterm birth, stillbirth, and low birth weight. During extreme weather events like hurricanes or wildfires, there are the direct injuries from the catastrophe but also increased incidence of domestic violence and child abuse. When the power goes out, people can die of heat stroke without air-conditioning. Warmer, wetter weather means increased spread of mosquito-borne illnesses. When the remnants of Hurricane Ida hit New York City in 2021, people living in substandard basement apartments drowned in the floodwater.

When the center doesn't hold, it shows up in myriad nightmarish ways, and it shows up first on and in the bodies of the most vulnerable. The fact that climate disasters are first primarily hitting marginalized people—people whose voices are often unheard—means some of us may not understand what is coming until it is way too late. But nurses *are* noticing.

Back in the 1990s, something strange happened: thousands of previously healthy, relatively young people in El Salvador and Nicaragua started turning up with end-stage kidney failure. They were mostly agricultural workers, people who labored on hot, humid, low-lying sugarcane plantations. They didn't have typical risk factors for kidney disease, and yet, they were dying from kidney failure in large numbers, and no one knew why. In the years since, kidney disease has become one of the leading causes of death in El Salvador, just barely behind heart disease. It is killing tens of thousands of people.

Then researchers around the world realized that something similar was happening to farmworkers in parts of South Asia. In some towns in Sri Lanka, nearly a quarter of the population has unexplained kidney disease. Other pockets of the illness have popped up in other very hot regions, like parts of Africa and the Middle East.

At first, scientists hypothesized that increased use of pesticides might be the cause, or heavy metal pollution in water, but pesticides and pollution are problems all over the world. It has become increasingly clear that this epidemic has two distinct components: hard outdoor labor plus increasingly extreme heat and humidity. When one of those factors is absent, so is this kind of kidney failure. For instance, in Nicaragua, workers in high-altitude coffee-growing villages, where temperatures are generally lower, generally do not have kidney failure, even though they work with pesticides. But in the lower, hotter areas, a threshold had slowly been crossed between what was survivable and what was not.

Since 1880, average global temperatures have risen by two degrees Fahrenheit, and humidity has increased, too. There is about 10 percent more moisture in the air now than in 1970. That might not seem like a lot, but your body knows the difference: the combination of heat and humidity makes it more difficult for your body to cool itself. Heat-related illness—when your body temperature rises to the level of a fever—causes the slow but certain breakdown of organ systems. As this happens, you might feel nauseated, weak, confused, and trembly. If the condition is left untreated, your body temperature will continue to rise; you may stop sweating altogether, or vomit. A body temperature of 104 degrees Fahrenheit or higher is classified as heat stroke, which can be fatal. But even if it doesn't get to that point, chronic heat-related illness can cause severe health problems, like kidney failure. If you spend all day outside in ninety-degree heat with high humidity, without regular access to shade, water, and rest, it can slowly, over the course of years, kill you.

This mysterious kidney failure is in the United States now, too—striking farm workers in hot, humid climates.

In the summers of 2018 and 2019, seventy-eight agricultural workers in Florida went to work in fields and plant nurseries wearing some unusual gear. Some of them wore a special cooling vest under their clothes, with ice packs embedded in it. Some wore a damp, cooling bandana around their necks. Some wore both the bandana and the vest, and some wore nothing but their regular clothes. All had swallowed a small pill that made its way through their digestive tract all day, where it measured their core body temperature. As the men and women worked, some noticed they were experiencing fewer heat symptoms than usual. At the end of the study, the group wearing the damp bandanas, which are cheap and widely available, had the least likelihood of a core body temperature exceeding thirty-eight degrees Celsius, the threshold at which heat-related illness begins. Research of this kind had never been done in the United States before.

The nurse behind this study was Roxana Chicas, PhD, RN, a scientist at Emory University. Chicas and her colleagues conduct research aimed at illuminating the connections among farmworkers' kidney problems, heat-related illness, and the lack of workplace protections. Their work is urgent: According to their research, 33 percent of farmworkers sustain acute kidney injury on any given workday, and the odds of kidney injury increase by 47 percent for every five-degree increase in the heat index. Add up enough acute kidney injuries and, eventually, kidneys start to fail.

But the misery of this epidemic is not fully conveyed by these numbers. There is a heartbreakingly simple way to slow or prevent this kidney failure, and it is regular access to water, rest, and shade—basic benefits that are not always provided by these workers' employers. Because many farmworkers are undocumented immigrants or asylum seekers, they are often unable or afraid to ask for safe working conditions. And when they do become ill, they may not be able to access health care. For Chicas, this is both unacceptable and personal.

Both of Chicas's parents were farmworkers in El Salvador, but her mother was forced to leave for the safety of the U.S. during El Salvador's Civil War, in which young women and children were routinely kidnapped. One of Chicas's first memories is from 1986, when she was four years old. She was clinging to her mother as they crossed the Rio Grande. "I remember crossing the river, and she had me on her shoulders. People would offer to help her carry me, and she always declined because she was so afraid that someone would kidnap me," Chicas said.

The two ended up in Georgia, where Chicas's mother supported them through housekeeping. Chicas, who has since become a U.S. citizen, became adept at moving among worlds: She grew up American, helping her mother navigate places where Spanish wasn't spoken. She was drawn to caring for others, and as a young adult, she went to nursing school and then didn't stop until she got her PhD. She had never imagined this kind of academic life was possible for her, but she started to ask herself why *not* her? She loved the work. When it came time to choose a dissertation topic, she didn't have a research question in mind, but she did have a community in mind: she wanted to work with immigrants from Latin America.

It was a stroke of luck that Chicas's PhD adviser, now her colleague, Linda A. McCauley, PhD, RN, was the primary investigator on the only longitudinal research study on the impact of heat on farmworkers' health in the United States. "It was a logical thing for me to do as an immigrant," Chicas said. "There's this huge shadow workforce. I felt like I wanted to honor that sacrifice that not only my mom, but also thousands of other immigrants have made, to come to this country and work backbreaking jobs to provide their kids the opportunity for a better life. This is where I was meant to do research."

I met Chicas at the Farmworker Association of Florida office in Apopka, where she was collecting the final data for a study tracking workers' kidney function as it related to heat over two years through the analysis of blood and urine samples and tracking the weather. Staff at the Farmworker Association are co-investigators, and the research is conducted at its offices because it is a place the workers know and trust and where their participation is kept confidential. (Their employers may not be supportive of research that implicates working conditions.) Other services are built into these data-collection days, like access to a food pantry.

If the old cliché is "canary in the coal mine," a more apt cliché for the future might be "laborer in the strawberry field." Or "worker in the fernery"—a term I learned from Chicas. Ferns are one of the big agricultural crops in the area; a nearby town calls itself the Fern Capital of the World, referring to the spray of anonymous greenery that comes with every bouquet of roses. I had never given the ferns a second thought, but they do not magically show up at the florist. They start out in vast fields covered with black plastic awnings. These tarps protect the plants, but they make the conditions much, much worse for the workers who pick the ferns. If it is ninety-five degrees Fahrenheit outside the awning, it is even hotter inside. The ferns grow to about hip high, so, to cut them, workers must stay bent over at the waist as they make their way down a row. They are paid $0.32 per bunch, for a total of $50 to $120 a day, depending on how fast they can pick. "In our data, we can see how much harder and faster they are working," Chicas said, comparing the per-piece workers to workers who are paid an hourly wage. "Their core body temperature is higher. They push themselves more than the hourly workers. Some of them go in at four a.m. with a headlamp, so they can work longer, pick more. Their bosses say they can take as many breaks as they want, but in reality, when they are making so little, many forgo any breaks. For something so trivial, they are working so hard. I can't see a bouquet the same way ever again."

Agricultural workers are twenty times more likely to die of heat stroke than the general population. And increasing heat has ramifications for other outdoor laborers, like construction workers, mail carriers, and utility workers. Construction workers, who have slightly better workplace protections than farm workers, are still thirteen times more likely to die from heat stroke than the general population. As the temperature continues to increase, anyone who works outside in the heat is at risk. Chicas's work is focused on proving the connection between increasing heat and humidity and farmworker health and on preventing those health problems as we move into a hotter future. This includes research on tools like the cooling bandana and advocacy for evidence-based changes to working conditions.

One might assume that employers in the United States *have* to provide basics like water and breaks, but the Occupational Safety and Health Administration (OSHA) only *recommends* that agricultural workers get these things. There are no federal workplace laws to enforce this. California and Oregon are the only states with permanent laws that mandate that growers provide these protections; Washington State has temporary emergency laws in effect. Oregon did not yet have its law in place during the summer 2021 heatwave, when Sebastian Francisco Perez was moving irrigation pipes at Ernst Nursery and Farms in St. Paul, Oregon. He collapsed and died of heat stroke. The temperature that day was over one hundred degrees Fahrenheit.

If Chicas and her colleagues can prove that people in this

community are being harmed and even killed by the combination of the warming climate and their work, and that this can be prevented with certain protections, then maybe legislators will force growers to provide those protections. But even in the absence of legislation, Chicas's work is vital to getting the word out to the workers about ways they can protect themselves.

This is what brought Chicas to the conference room at the Farmworker Association of Florida in the summer of 2021, warmly greeting the women and men participating in her studies. Like many nurses, she moved swiftly and efficiently, wearing sneakers. She was collecting data not only for the larger two-year study tracking workers' kidney functioning, but also for two smaller pilot studies. One measured whether drinking five liters of water with electrolytes protects farmworkers from heat illness better than drinking five liters of water alone. (It does.) The other pilot study was in collaboration with Georgia Tech: participants were testing a wearable nano device that could accurately measure core body temperature, heart rate, and other vitals throughout the day. These devices are easy to hide under a shirt, whereas other ways of measuring core body temperature are clunkier and potentially noticeable. The swallowable sensor, for instance, also requires that the worker carry something that looks like a cell phone from 1998.

As Chicas met with each worker, speaking in Spanish, she gave them a health snapshot, pulled from their on-site blood and urine analysis: their vitals, average blood sugar, hydration, cholesterol, markers of kidney function. She listened to their questions and let them know which results might need follow-up.

She does this because she is determined that the participants get something immediate and tangible from participating in the study. She gathers their health information not just for her data, but also for *them*, so that these twice-yearly data collection visits are more like miniature physicals. Often, she is the only health care provider they see regularly.

The walls of the conference room are covered in poster-size printouts of the studies that emerged from the data collected here. The information, Chicas said, belongs to this community and not in an academic journal behind a paywall. This is not typically the way research is done, but Chicas is also not a typical researcher: she is an immigrant herself, committed to climate justice, and she is a nurse grounded in nursing's person-centered ethos. If these perspectives were more common in researchers, perhaps research would be different.

That afternoon, Chicas was particularly worried about one participant, a woman who worked at a nearby plant nursery. Chicas swabbed the woman's fingertip with alcohol and pricked it, drawing a drop of blood to check her A1C, a blood sugar measurement. The woman had uncontrolled diabetes, and Chicas had been trying to help her get the medication she needed.

While Chicas processed the woman's blood sample, Nezahualcoyotl Xiuhtecutli, PhD, the general coordinator of the Farmworker Association and a co-investigator, sat with the woman. He asked her a series of standardized questions about her day: *Do you think you were exposed to pesticides? Was there shade? What physical activities did you do at work today? Did you have a headache? Did you vomit? Feel confused? Do you have pain when peeing? How many times did you pee today?*

Those questions answered, Chicas sat next to the woman. "Is it okay if I give results here?" she asked her in Spanish, gesturing to the busy room. The woman agreed, and Chicas began. She explained that the woman's heart rate, blood pressure, and cholesterol were fine. Her kidneys were functioning normally now, though she was dehydrated all day. But there was no protein in her urine, which was good news for her kidneys.

"Your blood sugar level is lower than it was in January—when did you start taking the medication?" Chicas asked. The woman responded, and Chicas listened. "Are you taking it regularly, as you are supposed to? I recommend you put an alarm on your phone. Because it *is* helping. A little bit. It would be better if you take it every day." The woman responded to the effect that she felt fine. "It's normal not to have symptoms," Chicas told her. "We call it 'silent.' But in the long term, if you don't take care of it, the problems can be dangerous."

Later, Chicas was still worried about this woman. She told me that her next investigation would be into how heat illness affected farmworkers' ability to metabolize sugar. The workers are on their feet doing strenuous work all day, and yet, most are not metabolically fit. It's a puzzle, Chicas said, and she suspects heat stress may have something to do with it.

The human body is a porous organism. Our health is interconnected with everyone and everything around us. This understanding is part of a nursing perspective, and that interconnectedness is increasingly obvious: We breathe smoke, we choke. We work in hundred-degree heat, we get heatstroke. We drink lead-contaminated water, we are poisoned. Our neighbor is sick, we might soon be sick, too. The understanding of this interconnectedness—not in a spiritual sense, but in the most concrete and literal sense imaginable—is not new, and it's especially not new to nursing.

In the twelfth century, a nun-mystic-healer named Hildegard of Bingen conceptualized this environmental reality in extraordinary writings on health. Hildegard likely learned about the workings of the human body while running the infirmary at her monastery. A practical knowledge of the medications of her time is evident in her books *Causes and Cures* and *Physica*. Some of the remedies are fantastical, like a cure for leprosy that involves the liver of a unicorn ground with egg yolk to make an ointment. But others seem like they might actually work: "If one suffers in his head, so that his head is stuffy, and it is as if he were deaf, he should eat cloves often, and that stuffiness in his head will diminish."

But beyond those remedies, her theories on health are sweeping and gorgeous. One of her most striking images is of the human body reflecting the cosmos and the cosmos reflecting the human body, the big echoing the small and the small echoing the big. She writes, "The firmament contains stars just as a man has veins that hold him together . . . Just as veins traverse the whole body, from the heart to the head, so stars pass through the firmament. In the same way blood is moved in the veins and moves the veins, making them leap and giving them a pulse, so fire is moved in the stars and causes them to be moved and to emit sparks."

For Hildegard, life was defined by a green force she called *viriditas*, universal in people, animals, and plants. *Viriditas* is a spiritual idea but also a literal one, grounded in the physical realities Hildegard saw all around her. She lived in an agricultural society, and the cycles of birth, growth, and death were obvious to her, inescapable even, as life depended on the ability to raise plants and animals. Her theories of human health revolved around *tending*, almost as in farming. She took the then-standard idea of the humors and matched them to natural elements, like air and water. Any imbalance in those environmental inputs, she believed, could stifle *viriditas*, working similarly in a fish or an herb or a person. The thing that *was* life was possible only when the environmental elements were in balance. Hildegard was not the only one to spin a theory like this; similar ideas exist in other cultures. These very old and completely sensical ideas about interconnection speak directly to nursing today.

The interconnectedness of all natural systems, all *life*, is a scientific reality nursing can address. Teddie M. Potter, PhD, RN, directs the Planetary Health program at the University of Minnesota School of Nursing. "I think we have forgotten our membership in the natural system," Potter said. "We've forgotten that we belong. We're a member in this system, and the system affects us in ways that affects all members of the system." She continued: "So, consider a plant. Whether it has adequate water, what's the nature of its soil, and is it exposed to sunshine? That determines whether that plant grows or doesn't survive. Why would we think we're any different?"

Potter argues that nurses have a crucial role to play as we all grapple with multisystem failure on earth. "There's a lot of grief and kind of a sense of 'Is it all done? Is the story already written? We're not going to make it.' But it's about helping nurses rise to our leadership role. We have always been the ones to say, 'There's something more we can do.'" That is exactly what makes nurses natural leaders against climate change: Nurses know all about the porousness of the human body. They notice problems before anyone else. And they know there's always something more that can be done—mitigation, comfort, advocacy, problem solving—even when there's no clear fix.

Christy Haas-Howard, MPH, RN, is engaged in this fight as someone who knows the particular horror of watching a child struggle to breathe. All three of her children have asthma, and she's a school nurse in Denver, where, at some public schools, 20 to 30 percent of all kids have the disease, which in rare cases can be fatal. Asthma rates are increasing in all populations, but especially in children, and the increase has been linked to increasingly bad air quality, which comes with climate change.

Haas-Howard told me a story about a Colorado school nurse who went outside during wildfire season and saw kids having football practice while ash was falling from the sky. The nurse asked the coach about it, and he said it was fine because they were monitoring the air quality—but from a sensor in an entirely different part of the county.

"The school nurse was like, 'Open your eyes! There is ash falling from the sky!'" Haas-Howard said. They ended the practice.

Sometimes a nurse's job is to emphatically state the obvious, but as Haas-Howard argues, each school should have a reliable way to test real-time, on-site air quality. It's the kind of thing everyone needs to check, like the weather. And for school nurses, it's part of keeping kids safe.

In 2018, Haas-Howard worked with the Denver Department of Public Health and Environment to establish an initiative called Love My Air, so that Denver schools could respond in real time to air quality, which is often dangerously bad. Through the program, forty schools have air quality sensors, and they use the data in multiple ways. When a child has an asthma attack, the school nurse can immediately check the air quality, to see if that might have been the trigger, and help the child better manage their asthma going forward. The existence of this data has led the kids to want to take action, too: a group of elementary students saw that the air quality at their school declined at pick-up and drop-off, as parents let their car engines idle as they waited in the parking lot, so they decided they needed to institute a no-idling policy.

Jessica LeClair, MPH, RN, has also seen climate change impact children's ability to breathe, not because of air quality but because of flooding and mold. In 2011, she was working at Public Health Madison and Dane County, in Wisconsin, when, at a neighborhood meeting, a school principal raised concerns that he was seeing more kids with asthma than ever before. The families were at that meeting, and they said they thought they knew why: Their apartments had never recovered from major flooding going back to 2008 and from repeated flooding since then. Their basements, they said, were filled with mold, so landlords had boarded them up. But now the mold was creeping up the vents, and their children were having trouble breathing.

LeClair said she had a terrible moment of realization that this was a multilayered emergency: the neighborhoods most affected were communities of color, recent immigrants. They were afraid to bring the problems up to their landlords or to building inspectors, fearing eviction. Also, every time the area flooded again, kids played in the waters, which were filled with dangerous pollutants. In Madison, the nights are warming faster than the days, making for hotter nights than ever before, which can also lead to asthma attacks.

First, LeClair went to a stormwater engineer for the city and explained that this neighborhood was having problems with flooding, that it was causing asthma in children. He told her that the flooding was particularly bad because of the water level in the nearby lake, but the lake was under state control, and there was nothing his office could do. The state was more concerned about keeping lakefront property owners happy than about dealing with flooding in poorer neighborhoods.

For seven years, LeClair tried to get the city public health department to do something—to act on climate change, to mitigate the health impacts that were already happening. And for seven years, she heard things like "We're just a small city. What can *we* do about climate change?" And "Why are you, *a nurse*, trying to take on climate change?" They thought it wasn't her lane. Undaunted, LeClair, together with a few colleagues, compiled a climate and health report, often working on her own time, unpaid. The public health department refused to publish it.

"I pushed and I pushed and I pushed and I pushed," LeClair said. "I pushed to not only do the assessment on the health effects of climate change in Madison Dane County, but then to create a plan in capacity and infrastructure, like other departments are doing around the country. They *would not do it*. And this is what it came down to: paying for my time *as a nurse*. So, not really understanding climate change, but then also not seeing *how* this is nursing," she said. "You don't have to change my job title to have me do this work. This is *absolutely* within my scope."

She wanted to assess a health problem, make a plan, and then implement that plan—that's what nurses do. But too many people don't understand what nurses do. In the end, LeClair had to leave the public health department in order to work toward climate justice. She became an instructor at the University of Wisconsin School of Nursing, at Madison: "I want to build up the future nursing workforce so that more nurses demand this kind of work and more nurses understand that this *is* nursing." After LeClair left, the public health department finally published the report she'd produced. What if LeClair had been given the resources she needed to tackle the problem? And what if the people controlling the budgets actually understood nursing practice, training, and scope? There might be fewer children struggling to breathe in Madison.

Katie Huffling, DNP, RN, knows that people don't always think of nurses as being on the front lines of climate change. As the executive director of the Alliance of Nurses for Healthy Environments, she brings nurses to Capitol Hill to tell lawmakers how climate change is hurting people now and to lobby for policies to address it. She sees it as a completely natural role for nurses, part of a long tradition of environmental nursing that includes Hildegard of Bingen and Florence Nightingale.

Huffling describes how climate change is affecting even the most everyday tasks nurses do, like planning a patient's discharge from the hospital. Air-conditioning, for instance, is now a necessary health intervention for the elderly and people with respiratory or cardiac disease. So, upon their discharge, their nurse will need to determine: Do they have a reliable air conditioner? Can they pay their electricity bill? Will the electricity grid hold up? Sometimes, of course, the answers to these questions is no. People don't always have what they need in order to be safe. That's where policy must come in. Huffling says legislators will need to expand Medicaid and Medicare to include coverage for expenses like electricity and air-conditioning. "It's way cheaper to keep someone at home than have them keep being readmitted to the hospital," she pointed out.

In 2022 at Emory University, Roxana Chicas was analyzing her data from Florida, and she found the results devastating. Over the course of two years, the participating workers' kidney function deteriorated dramatically. In their first visit, 15 percent of the workers had developed an acute kidney injury during a workday. Two years later, 27 percent of the same workers had developed an acute kidney injury on any given workday. There was also a marked decrease in how well the workers' kidneys filtered waste overall.

"We were expecting to see some decline," Chicas said. "I would say that this is more than I expected. It's almost a third of the workers, which is striking and concerning. I think that this has a lot to do with heat exposure and climate change. And I think that everyone now is at risk." I asked her what this meant for the workers, and she pointed out that many of them wouldn't be able to get care because they were undocumented and that, even if they did go back to their home country, dialysis would be hard to come by in those places. There was a long pause. "I think it means loss of life," she said. We were talking about young people, mothers and fathers, people who were hoping their kids might have a chance to become someone like Chicas.

Chicas and her colleagues will continue to try to answer these questions, to give the information to the people who need it, to try to prevent loss of life in any way they can. Now that they know, for instance, that electrolytes work, they are going to determine exactly which electrolytes are best and in what quantity, and then they'll get that word out to the affected workers. Of course, the situation will only grow more urgent: climate change and the food supply chain and migration come together in a web of complications that will reach everyone. "Climate change is a big driver of migration. And these are two issues that have to be resolved for the planet and for humanity," Chicas said. "And I'm hoping our research contributes to that. Me being a nurse and an immigrant and a scientist—I'm trying to showcase that. Because nurses are trained to look at things holistically. Nurses see things."

CHAPTER 8

ADDICTION

Staying Alive: How Radical Acceptance Can
Transform Substance Use Care

Jason Fox, NP, is a nurse practitioner specializing in addiction at Boston Medical Center (BMC). He leans forward as he speaks, smiles often, and even over Zoom, his demeanor suggests an openness that is almost startling in its sincerity. The people he cares for are often in the hospital for weeks at a time, and some come back again and again, suffering from severe medical problems that follow from drug and alcohol addiction.

"I say to them, 'I'm happy you're here; I'm happy you are safe,'" Fox said. I could tell that he meant it—and I could imagine what a relief it might be for his patients to hear it. Because Fox's genuine concern is not necessarily the norm among those who care for people with substance use disorder. Instead, providers sometimes treat people struggling with addiction as a burden or, in dismissive emergency room parlance, "frequent fliers," and their problems as personal moral failures. But this stigma has profound life-or-death consequences: If someone has been treated badly at a hospital in the past, they may be less likely to seek treatment when they need it. "Patients are waiting literally until they absolutely can't wait anymore to come to the hospital," Fox said. "Unfortunately, by the time they come in, they may need intensive care."

But there's a more humane and effective alternative: How differently might a patient experience the hospital if their nurse was genuinely happy to see them, exactly as they are? And what if that nurse was trained to help a patient think about their substance use and define their own goals for treatment? The care Fox provides is rooted in harm reduction, a model that revolves around the idea that people are autonomous and worthy of safety whether they are using substances or not. This framework, a kind of radical acceptance, doesn't start from an assumption that people can be, want to be, or even should be abstinent. Instead, it prioritizes any healthful change that minimizes the negative consequences of substance use. This goes against the long-established norm that the only valid goal in addiction treatment is total abstinence.

Hospitalization is an opportunity for nurses to intervene in someone's life in many ways—not just in the acute problem that brought them to the hospital. In fact, many patients welcome a nurse's intervention in regards to their substance use. A 2012 study found that 95 percent of hospital patients were comfortable with their bedside nurse discussing alcohol use with them and offering referrals to treatment if necessary. But not all *nurses* are comfortable with or adept at talking about substance use disorder or offering care for it. Some carry judgment or fears they need to manage, or they may simply believe that addiction is not in their purview, as it is not often dealt with in nursing education. That's why Fox not only sees patients himself, but also runs a fellowship for bedside nurses at BMC that provides training in harm reduction interventions. These can involve teaching patients about safer ways to inject, understanding that agitated behavior might mean poorly treated withdrawal, or even just being comfortable asking questions about substance use and listening without judgment. The hope is that, someday, this will mean that every patient who comes into BMC with a substance use problem will get a nurse who is ready and able to respond in a helpful way. This is increasingly important as alcohol- and drug overdose–related deaths continue to rise, and are higher now than ever before.

The permanent BMC addiction team consists of Fox and other nurse practitioners, a social worker, a recovery advocate, and an attending physician. Students and fellows rotate in and out. Fox is called to all parts of the hospital, as addiction touches everyone: He might go from seeing a woman in labor and delivery; to a patient in the ICU after a car crash; to the ER, where someone is in alcohol withdrawal; to a medical floor where someone is on six weeks of intravenous antibiotics for a bone infection following intravenous drug use. Fox also helps other clinicians understand how a patient's substance use might affect their care. "I'm telling the medicine team or the surgical team which medications to order, how we're going to go up on doses, and leading that charge," he said. "Part of the work is educating *them* about addiction because, unfortunately, that does affect patient care."

When Fox meets a patient, he tries to read the room: He identifies himself right away as being a nurse from the addiction team. He sits down as soon as he can, instead of standing over the patient. If the room lights are off, he leaves them off. He speaks in a quiet voice if the patient is quiet. He asks, "How are you?" Again, he really means it. And he's not afraid to use humor to lighten the mood. "Patients are not used to genuineness," he said. "If you're uncomfortable, the patient is going to know you are uncomfortable."

Fox says he likes to think of his job as bringing a tray of options to the patient and letting them choose what is best for them. Often the most pressing concern is withdrawal: it must be treated correctly, or it will be unbearable, and the patient might leave the hospital and not get the care they need. As Fox gets to know the patient over the course of a hospitalization, he asks them to think about making a plan—he tells them it has to be *their* plan, not his. What are their goals?

One goal might be getting off substances entirely, and Fox can help them find abstinence-based treatment programs or 12-step groups. But other people might have different goals: they might want to know how to prevent skin problems from injecting, or how to avoid reusing needles. Fox talks to patients about safer injecting techniques, such as avoiding dangerous spots like the neck and groin. He asks where they are getting their needles and tells them about safe needle exchange programs. He can start patients on maintenance medications like methadone, to help them get off heroin. And, in the last several years, he's been talking a lot about fentanyl, which is more potent than heroin and can cause an overdose quickly. He tells patients to carry Narcan with them, and to try to use with a friend, with a phone nearby. In these ways, his practice of harm reduction acknowledges that drug and alcohol use is a reality and seeks to minimize the problems wrought by addiction.

"Patients with opioid disorder that are on methadone maintenance treatment or buprenorphine maintenance—just by being on the medication, they have a fifty percent decreased risk of overdose death," he said. "So, when we talk about lifesaving medications, those medications truly are. And we really do view the treatment of substance use disorder like any other chronic disease or illness, whether it's diabetes or heart failure."

Of course, the wider world does not always think of substance use this way, and resources are scarce. There's often not enough of anything to go around—most crucially, beds at inpatient substance use treatment programs. When a patient is ready to be discharged, and they'd like to go to inpatient treatment, it can be wrenching to tell them that's not possible. Fox explains: "It's like an eclipse. The day of discharge has to match up with an open treatment bed. And many of the treatment centers, they are worried that the patients going are going to be difficult to care for, that they're medically unstable." That's why many substance use treatment centers won't take people straight from the hospital. But then, where do they go, and what happens to them?

As I listened to Fox describe this dense thicket of logistics, an old knot twisted in my stomach. I knew most of this already, though I had tried to forget it: My father, who lived in Massachusetts, struggled with substance use his whole life, as well as with mental illness and major physical illness, including Crohn's disease and hepatitis C. He'd be discharged from the hospital willing to go to treatment, but often there were no beds, or no beds for someone like him. I suppose there must be a population of people with severe substance use disorder who are in otherwise perfect health, but I haven't met them. What I knew back then was that all these hurdles told me exactly how little my father's survival mattered to the system—or, more to the point, how little his survival was *expected*. As he bounced in and out of the hospital, sometimes I felt he was seen as the walking dead.

I remember thinking, in the years he was dying, that there had to be a better way, that there had to be *someone* who could look at his entire self: at both his genuine need for pain pills and his abuse of pain pills; at his sincere desire to get treatment and his seeming inability to be abstinent; at his attachment to living alone in his own apartment and his inability to keep himself safe. I wasn't looking for a magical fix; I was looking for mitigation. I was looking for a health care professional to see my father, *really see* him. I knew my father was not likely to change, but I couldn't accept that there was *nothing* anyone could do to help. But there was no way, within the health care system as I understood it then, to ask those questions: *What would be best for him? How can we help him as he is, where he is?* And there was no one to ask. But, talking to Fox, I finally understood what I had been looking for—whom I had been looking for.

Harm reduction in the United States has its roots in activist movements: community health programs started by the Black Panthers and the Young Lords, and needle exchange programs started by HIV/AIDS activist groups like ACT UP (AIDS Coalition to Unleash Power), when it became clear that intravenous drug use was one way the virus that caused AIDS was spreading. The needle exchange programs were based on those already established in Europe, but they were at first either illegal or in a kind of legal limbo in the United States. These programs dovetailed with other innovations, such as the development of maintenance medications like methadone for opioid addiction, which began in the 1970s.

The moralizing idea underpinning the so-called war on drugs was, and in many ways still is, that if you used drugs, you deserved any consequences that flowed from that. This brutal framework was designed to throw people away, particularly Black and brown people, and it certainly has not reduced rates of substance use disorder. Harm reduction is a refusal of all that. It insists on the agency and autonomy of people who use drugs and alcohol. Once substance use is accepted as a reality, once people are valued no matter what, the question becomes what are the ways to lessen the harms of drug use, both to the individual and to their community?

For family members of those with addiction, or for those who have succeeded in abstinence, this approach can be hard to accept. But not everyone wants to be or can be abstinent, and survival can be a process that changes over time. The wish that abstinence would work for everyone with substance use disorder is a wish for a different world. Meanwhile, what we have been doing isn't working.

Drug use and abuse has always existed, but the meanings of intoxication and what is considered socially acceptable and not have varied tremendously. The question of how to deal with the problem of addiction is a very old one, and there have always been those who advocated offering help that would reduce harm, not impose punishment. Sixteenth-century Persian physician Imad al-Din Mahmud wrote a book called *Afyunieh*, one of the first medical texts to address addiction. It describes opium's uses, both medicinal and recreational, and how to treat opium addiction. The author suggests three possible strategies: reducing the time between opium doses, slowly reducing the dose itself, or substituting a different intoxicant for the opium, such as poppy skin or henbane (a poisonous herb of the nightshade family), and then slowly tapering off that.

These strategies are all very familiar to L. Synn Stern, MPH, RN, who runs a walk-in clinic at OnPoint NYC, an overdose prevention center in East Harlem, New York. Called New York Harm Reduction Educators, her organization provides comprehensive health and social services to their clients, about 70 percent of whom are experiencing homelessness. It includes a consumption room, where clients can use their own drugs with clean supplies, and immediate medical care should they need it.

When I asked Stern for strategies people can use to improve their health even if they are still using, she ticked off a list: "You can switch to a longer-acting drug. You can change the route of administration. People who are struggling to find a vein can switch to booty bumping: rectal insertion. That lasts a lot longer; there's a time delay. And it can give people a break from injections," she said. (This is something Imad al-Din Mahmud suggested for Ramadan consumption of opium four hundred years ago.) "There are inpatient programs," Stern continued, "and even if you just go there to rest and eat—rest and eat! You're off the street for a while. You're off your feet for a while. You're out of the weather. Plan your next moves. And providing Suboxone is wonderful," she added, referring to the brand name for buprenorphine, which, like methadone, is a prescribed maintenance medication and is a safer substitute for heroin and other opioids.

Stern's small office, which doubles as the clinic, is in the New York Harm Reduction Educators' unassuming brick building, which often has a cluster of people outside, talking and smoking. One afternoon in March, the welcome area was bustling with people going in and out. The space was equipped with several desks for clients' use, computers connected to the internet, a TV, some comfy chairs, several stacked washer-dryers, and bathrooms with showers. At the time of my visit, an alcove that will one day be a pharmacy was under construction. Upstairs, there was a wellness center that provides acupuncture and massage, a detox program developed by the Young Lords, the radical Puerto Rican civil rights group.

At the end of the intake room was a line of eight or nine people waiting to be checked in at a long table before entering what is called the safer consumption room—"safer" for obvious reasons. One by one, each person approached the table, where the staff greeted them. They filled out paperwork acknowledging that they had used drugs before, understood the risks, would keep their own drugs, and use only their own drugs. They gave permission to the program to provide emergency medical services if necessary. They also disclosed which drug they were going to use that day, how they were going to use it, their drug use and overdose history, their housing situation, and where they would have used had they not been able to use at the clinic (say, in a park, a public restroom, a subway station, or at a residence). The staff get to know the people who come in on a regular basis, so, if someone usually comes once a day, but starts coming three times a day, they know to check in and find out if something's wrong. The same goes for when a client switches to a potentially more harmful drug.

On one level, it is strange to see illicit drug use so carefully documented and explicitly planned, but this is part of effective care for people with substance use disorder. After all, the worst harm of substance use is death, and people are much more likely to survive doing drugs when they can do them in this consumption room or at its sister site in Washington Heights. Opened in late 2021, these two overdose prevention centers are the first legal programs of their kind in the United States. In the first four months they were open, the staff served nearly 1,000 clients and used Narcan to reverse 226 overdoses that would likely have been fatal in any other setting.

The consumption room is staffed by harm reduction specialists who have received training from Stern. One of them is Alsane Mezon, a petite woman with purple cat's-eye glasses and a forthright, friendly demeanor. She showed me around the room, pointing out the eight cubicles whose chairs face the wall, almost like library carrels. Each cubicle has a mirror on the wall side, so that the harm reduction specialists can see clients' faces, to make sure they are not falling unconscious, and the people using the cubicles directly face a mirror as they inject, snort, or swallow their drug—which seems like it might feel strange. There are also two bathrooms with heavy-duty fans and ventilation, where people can go for fifteen-minute increments to smoke their drug.

"You consume what you bring in. Otherwise, I bar you for the day," Mezon said, enforcing the rule on no exchange of drugs. She has both an innate warmth and the steely air of someone who is surprised by absolutely nothing. "Hi, honey!" she called out to someone as they entered the room.

Each person entering went through a series of steps: First, they visited the hand-washing station. Then they picked up the supplies they needed from neat caddies in the middle of the room. There were clean syringes and pipes, to use now or later, and portable sharps containers to go. Finally, the client sat at a cubicle to consume their drugs. If they wanted to, they could set up a folding privacy screen first. When I was there, only one of the seven people in the room had done so.

Mezon is there to make sure that if someone overdoses, they won't die. But she's also there for support and education. She pointed to a poster on the wall that showed photographs of the magnified tip of a needle: first, smooth, shiny, and sharp and, then, increasingly blunted and deformed. "That's what happens if you don't use a clean needle every time," she said. That's why people often get abscesses and skin infections, using old, blunt needles that tear the skin.

People can come into the clinic, use their drugs, and leave without much human interaction. But some people ask for help, and in that case, Mezon and the other harm reduction specialists step in. Mezon can't inject *for* them, of course, but she can advise them on the least risky ways to inject. She can explain that it will burn if they hit an artery. She can explain how to find a good vein, and she can help with a tourniquet. She can show someone how to use a fentanyl test to make sure their heroin is not cut with the more potent drug. She can make sure they are drinking enough water. And she can make sure they keep breathing and are well enough to leave the clinic. There are pulse oximeters to measure blood oxygen, a tank of oxygen and masks to supply it, and Narcan in both nasal spray and syringe form, which reverses opiate overdoses instantly.

She pointed out one young man who was standing in a cubicle with his foot up on a chair. The other harm reduction specialist, who is also an EMT, was bent next to him, helping tie a tourniquet. A trickle of blood was making its way down the man's leg, toward his white sneakers. "This young man would have been making a mess of himself," Mezon said. She said he comes in from Long Island to inject here. "So he can get home safe to his wife and kids. He wants it in his leg because he doesn't want his wife to see [tracks in] his arms."

It's obvious that Mezon loves the work, loves the people. "I'm a grandmother," she said. "I know that is someone's child. All I know is your mother wants you to come home, no matter who you are." She is a medical assistant by training, but she said she really wanted to be a nurse. I think she *is* a nurse, in any true sense of the word.

Stern comes into the safe consumption room when necessary, but she spends most of her time providing walk-in care in her office, at the other end of the hall. The current New York City government supports this program, and OnPoint is fully transparent about the services it provides. But safe consumption sites have been prevented from opening in other cities, like Philadelphia, and are in a kind of legal limbo outside New York. It's unclear how a state nursing board would regard the work. And so, there is an effort to separate, at least nominally, the official nursing work from the consumption room.

Stern came to this field in both a very direct and a highly improbable way. She was an activist in ACT UP and a community health worker, and before that, she was a sex worker who used drugs and experienced homelessness. She became a nurse in her forties. She has been exactly where her clients are now, and this background informs everything she does. "When I was homeless, I remember every nice touch I ever experienced," she said, sitting in her office. "You know, like this person who tied a scarf around my neck. That kind of thing would keep me going for months. And I want to be able to be *that* in someone's memory. My job is to just make them feel a little bit better when they leave. And if I can do that, I feel great."

When Stern first stopped using drugs, she was working at an inpatient treatment program based on the 12 Steps, a model that's grounded in the idea that substance use disorder is an incurable, progressive disease over which you have no control and that abstinence is the only acceptable outcome. Stern points out that 12-Step programs like Alcoholics Anonymous and Narcotics Anonymous can do a lot of good, in that they provide free, robust social support, which is no small thing. But she found herself philosophically opposed to the framework: It involved shaming, and there was little accommodation for relapse, which resulted in many people leaving and never coming back or, worse, internalizing the idea that they were powerless against the disease without learning any strategies to manage it. "It's either you're a hundred percent clean or you're just a failure and you start over and you're counting from day one again," she said, explaining how, with 12-Step programs, a relapse is thought to erase all the progress a person has made.

So, she left to work in community health. It was a time of tremendous need, the dawn of the AIDS epidemic, and she was galvanized by what she saw as friends died all around her, often unable to access care because of the stigma around the virus compounded by the stigma of being a drug user, or doing sex work, or being gay, or all the above. Around 1985, she started covertly giving out free syringes with other activists in New York City—first, on a small scale and, then, on a larger scale. These illegal peer-led programs would later become some of the first harm reduction programs in the city.

New York Harm Reduction Educators started out with a handful of ACT UP volunteers, Stern among them, doing syringe exchange in Harlem and the Bronx. They got the syringes shipped from a guy named Dave Purchase, who started exchanging clean needles for dirty ones in 1988 in Tacoma, Washington, from a little folding TV tray he set up on the sidewalk. He also handed out mittens, cookies, and condoms.

Syringe exchange programs worked: in the years after such programs were legalized in New York State, which was around 1992, HIV prevalence among people who used injected drugs fell from 50 percent to 17 percent. Stern continued to work in harm reduction and community health programs; she published in scholarly journals, and she wrote a detailed manual on health and safety measures for street sex workers, winkingly called *Tricks of the Trade*. But she became increasingly troubled by the substandard care she saw her friends and neighbors receiving from health care providers. She found herself wishing she had clinical skills, so she could step into that gap. That's when she went to nursing school.

"The big reason I became a nurse was I watched people get treated badly by health care providers, and I watched them die of things they shouldn't have died from. Completely preventable illnesses," she said. "Getting septic from a minor infection, or dying of pneumonias that weren't HIV-related. And being so afraid to go to the hospital because of their terrible experiences, delaying and delaying, until things were so widespread. And I just didn't want that to happen to people anymore." She became a nurse to alleviate the suffering she experienced and that she saw all around her. Nursing offers her a way to act on all she knows.

This is what brought her here—a nurse in her sixties now, with close-cropped gray hair and a steady, blue-eyed gaze, her compact frame in jeans. People often come to her office with multiple critical issues, some of which are intractable, the kind of health problems that follow from living on the street. Stern thinks about the aims of each encounter as twofold: "It's always, 'What does the person desperately want? Let me do that. And what's going on that might kill them? Let me do that, too.' So, trying to fit those things together and present it in such a way that it makes sense to them."

On that day, she had seen a woman who needed nursing care for multiple concerns. "She's like a hurricane," Stern said. "She has so many questions and so much anxiety, and she's in constant motion. And she's so dear and just so overwhelmed and so frightened." The woman was worried she had been exposed to HIV and hepatitis C. She had a cold sore she was worried about, too. "The usual anxieties of being small, female, drug-dependent, homeless, and hooking," Stern said. "Everything you can think of is happening to her all the time."

So, what did this woman want, and what did this woman need? Stern prescribed medication for a sexually transmitted disease, and she drew blood for labs, to test for other infections. In order to take the meds, the woman had to eat, but she didn't have any teeth. So, Stern, who had only a granola bar, went and found her something soft. She then checked the woman for lice and taught her how to use an insertive (or internal, or "female") condom; she was in a sexually abusive relationship, and she couldn't count on her partner to wear protection. She was very constipated, a common side effect of opioid use. For this, Stern taught her how to stick her thumb into her vagina and against the perineum to push out the feces that way. The woman decided to keep her meds at the overdose prevention center and come back every day to take them, so she wouldn't lose them, have them stolen, or be tempted to take them all at once. "That was a good decision on her part," Stern said.

Stern's nursing is very pragmatic, grounded in the unforgiving realities of life on the street. The next patient she saw was a man who hadn't been by for a long time. The last time she saw him, she told him she thought his leg was broken and that he should go to the hospital. It turned out she was right, but because he'd been treated so badly in hospitals before, he had delayed going, and he was embarrassed to tell her. By the time he went, his broken leg had become infected, and he needed surgery and a complicated skin graft. He was now in a wheelchair, homeless, and recovering from all that.

Stern spent a lot of time with him, talking to him about what had happened, making sure the infection was healing. She replaced his bandage with a fresh one, but he had to continue to keep the wound clean and his foot elevated. Stern had a few suggestions: He could sit on the sidewalk, put his foot on the chair, and hold onto the chair.

He could come to the clinic every day and go to the wellness center, where they have nice reclining chairs. He could also accept a bed in a nursing home, but Stern found that option unlikely. "But if he does any of those things, even a little bit, it's going to improve the circumstances," she said.

When harm reduction was new, in the 1970s and '80s—when Stern was getting boxes of syringes in the mail and giving them out uptown—basically any way to help people struggling with addiction that wasn't punitive or abstinence-based was illegal or made extraordinarily difficult. Syringe exchanges, Narcan use, the distribution of free condoms, opioid maintenance medications, fentanyl test strips, decriminalizing marijuana—all these have increasingly become an accepted part of public health practice over the last thirty-odd years. Now the Biden administration's official policy on drug overdose prevention is centered on harm reduction measures. In Canada, harm reduction has recently been taken even further: in an effort to protect people from street drugs cut with fentanyl, providers can prescribe opioids for people to use as they wish, to prevent the accidental overdoses that are so common now.

The increasing prevalence of harm reduction practice is good news. The evidence has shown that these measures really do save and improve lives. There are many reasons for the slow bend away from the punitive and ineffective war on drugs and toward more humane practices, including the utter relentlessness of people like Stern. But it's also important to note that the increased acceptance of harm reduction has coincided with a change in the "face" of substance use—from Black and urban to white and suburban or rural. Substance use disorder doesn't vary much along racial demographic lines—for instance, from 2015 through 2019, substance use disorder occurred in 7.8 percent of white people and 7.1 percent of both Black and Hispanic people, but overdose deaths of white Americans have sharply risen over the last decade. In other words, substance use affects everyone; what differs is how substance use in different communities is treated and understood by health care workers and law enforcement. Black, urban communities were devastated by the criminalization of substance use, but with the increased focus on the impact of substances on *white* communities, less punitive policies have gained acceptance. That's not a coincidence.

The nurses who try to reduce harm know about the vast injustices and sorrows of drug use in this country. That's why Jason Fox's mission to create more nurses who can operate this way is crucial: he's nursing his patients, but he's also trying to fundamentally change nursing's approach to people with substance use disorder. If he and others like him succeed, maybe radical acceptance and harm reduction won't be fringe anymore; maybe they will be the default. The nursing goal of meeting people where they are, and doing no harm, requires it.

"When patients do come back to the hospital, there's no shame, there's no judgment," Fox said. "We fall down, but we get back up. The focus is on the getting back up."

CHAPTER 9

COLLECTIVE

No Angels: Nursing as Labor

That the nurse is a worker, no one can deny.

—LAVINIA L. DOCK, RN

In 2004, California nurses went to war against Governor Arnold Schwarzenegger. The governor had just issued an emergency order halting a nurse-to-patient ratio law. The law, which is still the only of its kind in the country, specifies the maximum number of patients to whom a nurse can be assigned, with different ratios for different settings: one nurse to two patients in the ICU, for instance, or one nurse to five patients on a standard medical-surgical floor. The bill had been signed into law by the previous governor, but it was vociferously opposed by the California Hospital Association, which unsuccessfully sued to stop it. When Schwarzenegger came to office, under the banner of conservative fiscal responsibility, he halted full implementation of the bill, which then got tied up in court. Shortly after, nurse protestors interrupted one of the governor's speeches to unfurl a banner that read KEEP YOUR HANDS OFF OUR RATIOS, a reference to the multiple groping allegations against the governor. As the nurses were removed from the room, Schwarzenegger called them a "special interest group." He went on: "I'm always kicking their butt."

Unfortunately for him, the California Nurses Association (CNA) labor union was then led by a pugilistic former Teamster, RoseAnn DeMoro, and a core group of nurse labor leaders who had broken away from the American Nurses Association to become an organization that was not afraid to flex its power. And they knew that part of nurses' power lay in their position as advocates for the public, defenders of people when they were at their most vulnerable. "If you're a patient's advocate, you're advocating for that patient. You're not advocating for the profit of that hospital," DeMoro told NPR in 2006. When Schwarzenegger picked a fight with nurses, the CNA was ready to fight back, not just on the ratio law, but also on the need to be understood as the skilled and indispensable workers they are—to make it clear, once and for all, that if *any* of us hopes to be safe and well, nurses must be able to do their jobs.

For the next year, anywhere Schwarzenegger went, the nurses went, too. At every speech, every fund-raiser, there were nurses assembled out front, chanting and holding signs with slogans like PATIENTS ARE OUR SPECIAL INTEREST. They flew planes over his events trailing banners. They hired a jazz band to play a funeral dirge as they carried coffins to the State Capitol building. When Schwarzenegger held a Super Bowl party, they flew a blimp over his house. When he went to Boston for a Rolling Stones fund-raiser at Fenway Park, the CNA partnered with Massachusetts nurses to make such a commotion outside that Mick Jagger commented that, actually, he loved nurses. On Oscars Night, the CNA rented the hotel function room next to Schwarzenegger's gala, where they threw their own, very conspicuous party. They rented a bus and trailed Schwarzenegger all around the state with what they called the Truth Squad, a group of nurses along with Annette Bening and Warren Beatty, who lent their star power to combat Schwarzenegger's. The nurses also put the governor up for "auction" on eBay. Their campaign had a vehemence that approached glee. There was no peace for the governor; no matter where he went, furious nurses were there.

The fact that it was *nurses* who were deploying aggressive political theater was attention-getting in and of itself. In some circles, including among some nurses, it was seen as transgressive for nurses to engage in this kind of advocacy—the idea of what is "professional" has often been used as a cudgel to keep nurses quiet and to prevent them from organizing. But these protests were electric precisely *because* they challenged what it meant to be workers in a caring profession and *mostly women* workers in a caring profession. Gerard Brogan, RN, director of nursing practice at CNA and at its national partner, National Nurses United, remembers the efforts to turn nurses on to their own power. "We came across a lot of 'This is unprofessional; professionals do not unionize,'" he said. "I wasn't the only one, but I personally had a lot of meetings in people's houses to thrash through these arguments. It's entirely professional to be in a union. It's entirely professional to be in control of your own destiny."

The CNA was originally founded in 1903 as a branch of the American Nurses Association. But this affiliation caused increasing internal conflict, because the ANA wasn't focused on collective bargaining or organizing around nurse-to-patient ratio laws. "The ANA historically has been conservative. Just really buying into that idea that this is a woman-dominant profession, and we're handmaids to the medical authorities—that would be doctors and those who administrate hospitals," Brogan said. "They were firmly opposed to the ratio law because, frankly they're in cahoots with the industry."

So, in 1993, a core group of labor-minded nurses wrested away control of the organization and started challenging norms about how nurses should act. "The ANA did not want to build power," Brogan said. "I think the essential thing we did was that we changed the paradigm of the nursing organization to pursue power instead of prestige."

Health care in the 1990s was ripe for revolution, in the sense that things were very bad: the Clinton health care plan had failed spectacularly, and HMOs were on the rise, consolidating practices, denying benefits, requiring prior authorization for every little thing, and generally squeezing the system for all it was worth. Brogan says that nurse staffing, always a problem, was increasingly short, and nurses were struggling to care for high patient loads. He saw it himself as a charge nurse at the UCSF Health medical center.

After breaking from the ANA, the insurgent CNA immediately dedicated itself to the biggest issue for their members at the time: patient-to-nurse ratios. It took over a decade to get the ratio law passed, which involved unprecedented organizing within the nurse community but also reaching out to the public to make it clear that this was everyone's issue. "We aligned ourselves with the consumers of health care, not the deliverers of health care," says Brogan, who himself led a publicity initiative that CNA called "patient watch," sharing stories of patients who had had care denied. The PR campaign was designed to show what health care looked like when the hospital industry and HMOs made all the clinical decisions, instead of clinicians. Every day, he publicized the story of someone who had been failed by this system. One was an elderly man who called a Kaiser hospital in California complaining of chest pain. The man didn't meet Kaiser's bar to be admitted at that time. While he was on the phone, being told he wasn't sick enough to require inpatient care, he had a heart attack.

The nurses pointed to these draconian cost-cutting measures as part of a larger movement on the part of health care corporations to skimp on the costs of patient care—particularly, nurse staffing, replacing nurses with other workers without the same training who would be paid much lower salaries. Nurses reached out to the public to say, *We're in this together. The more nurses in hospitals, the safer you will be.* This was a tactic, but it was also true. Research suggests that the higher the level of nurse staffing in a hospital, the more likely you are to be discharged alive. The message was also based in a deeper, older ethical truth: the relationship between nurse and patient is and has always been the bedrock of good care. "The campaign was based on our relationship with the public," Brogan says. And "the public" is all of us—all of us with a fallible human body, all of us who have watched the body of someone we love fail and have worried about them getting the care they needed.

And so, in 2004, after the country's first and only nurse-to-patient ratio law was finally on the books, along came Arnold Schwarzenegger, glibly calling nurses a special interest group and issuing cynical emergency orders to stop the ratio law from going into effect. He probably thought the nurses would retreat meekly. He did not understand nurses as indispensable, knowledgeable workers with powerful connections to their communities.

When the war between the CNA and Schwarzenegger began, the governor's approval rating was 65 percent. By the time the nurses had finished with him, not only had they joined with teachers and firefighters to defeat three ballot propositions directed against public workers, but they had also beaten the governor in court so the ratio law could proceed as intended. His approval ratings had fallen into the 30s.

That victory was born of nurses not playing "nice," a quality that has often been demanded of them throughout history in order to silence them. These nurses were insisting on their status as professional

skilled workers, not as "professionalized" natural caregivers—
essentially, trained mothers who had duties, not rights, which was
how nurses had been treated and understood since Nightingale's
model took hold. It was an inversion of everything.

Hospital administrators have been trying to cut nursing costs
since the dawn of modern hospitals. In the United States, many of
the earliest nursing schools of the nineteenth to mid-twentieth centuries were run by hospitals, where the trainee nurses, all women,
lived and worked in a kind of apprenticeship program, though in-
struction was scarce. As historian Susan M. Reverby, PhD, observes
in her book *Ordered to Care*, "Autonomy was sacrificed and altruism
was sanctified . . . Nursing education was called training; in reality, it
was work." While the nurses were paid a small "allowance," they were
also hired out, and the hospitals collected and kept those fees, making the nurses' net cost to the hospitals close to zero. By around 1920,
eighteen hundred hospitals had schools of nursing whose trainees
provided most of the patient care essentially for free.

The hospitals' desire for trainee labor created a strangely divided
nursing workforce: Hospitals insisted there was a shortage of bedside
nurses and pressed their nursing schools to enroll more and more
students to provide that care. Meanwhile, when those students graduated, most of them could not get a job with a hospital, even if they
had wanted one. A nurse who trained at Boston City Hospital in 1920,
for instance, would have had no expectation that the hospital would
hire her when she graduated—because she now wanted payment and
better working conditions. So, most graduate nurses worked in what
was called "private duty," in which they were hired by individuals
who could afford them. This meant there was often an oversupply of
graduate nurses who worked privately, while hospitals continued to
insist there were not enough nurses—by which they meant nurses who
would work for free.

This completely self-created problem became only more acute as the number of hospitals and the complexity of medical care increased. Hospitals proposed various schemes, like creating a lesser-trained, lower-paid workforce to fill in the gaps. Variations on this idea have never gone away. Nurse educators proposed solutions like separating nurse education from nurse labor, thus producing better-educated and -prepared nurses whom the hospitals could hire. But this was not the kind of solution the hospitals had in mind. This impasse persisted for years, through various incarnations, until, very slowly, the concept of the graduate staff nurse employed at hospitals became more and more the norm.

In her book *Nursing the Nation*, nurse historian Jean C. Whelan, PhD, points out that this conflict over the expectation that nurses work out of the goodness of their hearts created an adversarial relationship that has persisted ever since. "Accustomed to using more pliant and obedient student workers," she writes, "hospitals approached nurses' reluctance to take on staff nurse work with punitive measures that worked to repel nurses rather than attract them to hospital employment."

As time passed, the devaluing of nurses only deepened because the insurance system, which is built around reimbursement for medicines and procedures, has hidden the true value of nursing work. Whelan puts it this way: "When hospitals finally did employ nurses in large numbers, they effectively hid the nursing costs in patient room-and-board costs they charged to insurers. . . . which obscured and devalued a service considered to be essential to modern health care." This remains true: Nurses are considered a hospital expense because their practice is usually not billable to insurance the way physicians' services are. If you are admitted to a general medical floor, you might share your nurse with four other patients, or with seven other patients. Regardless, the bill for your room and board will likely be the same. For the hospital, it is exponentially more profitable to have fewer nurses caring for more patients, but this financial interest is entirely contrary to what is best for the patient.

While hospitals say there is a shortage of nurses—which seems to be a forever condition—they largely reject the idea that fixable problems in nurses' working conditions could be the main cause. And hospital groups often insist they *can't* agree to better nurse-to-patient ratios or to higher levels of nurse staffing overall; there simply aren't enough nurses to hire, they insist. The California Hospital Association claimed they could not possibly find enough nurses to meet the ratio law's staffing requirements, and yet, when forced to do so, they did. The number of nurses with active licenses in California increased when the law went into effect, suggesting that trained nurses were already out there and were enticed to return to bedside care by the improved conditions, a concurrent rise in salaries, or both.

The truth of the famous nursing shortage—or staffing crisis, or pipeline problem, or vacancy issue—is all in how you look at it. It's not just one thing; it is many things. It is true that in many low-income rural areas, there are not enough nurses (or health care workers generally) to go around. And, as Patrick McMurray, MSN, RN, has pointed out, there is a true shortage of nurses from Black and brown and low-income communities, the very groups who have often been shut out of nursing. It's also true that nursing skews a bit older, and many Boomer nurses are retiring just as demand for nurses is increasing.

But the ever-present nationwide nursing shortage has never been about a simple lack of nurses. In fact, the National Academies of Sciences, Engineering, and Medicine forecasts that the nursing workforce will grow in the 2020s and that there is and will be no large nationwide shortage of nurses this decade. In the United States today, there are about 4.4 million currently licensed registered nurses. According to the U.S. Bureau of Labor statistics, only 3 million of them are currently employed in nursing, about 60 percent of those in inpatient hospitals. The nurses who don't work in hospitals may be employed in home care, outpatient offices, schools, clinics, in policy, or in other settings with better conditions. But some of those 4.4 million have retired early or walked away from the profession entirely. In fact, newly graduated nurses quit their jobs in their first and second years of work by rates of 30 to 57 percent. All this suggests that the big-picture problem is not a lack of nurses, but nurse turnover. Why do so many nurses leave bedside nursing or leave the profession altogether?

Nurses often suffer what is called a moral injury—when they have more patients than they can safely care for, and when they are forced to participate in a situation that goes against their deepest sense of what is right. This can be so excruciating that it causes them to quit the profession. And what is that like for patients?

I had an experience with my mother in the hospital that is embarrassing to tell. She was bedridden and had had a bowel movement in a bedpan. She was on a general medical floor, and her nurse clearly had more patients than she could care for. I asked the nurse if she could come in to help my mother clean up and remove the bedpan from under her, and the nurse told me we would have to wait: she was hustling to this bed, to that bed. There didn't seem to be a nursing assistant who could help. My mother was bony and had cancer that had spread to her vertebrae, so it was very painful for her to remain resting on the bedpan. Why didn't I move her myself? I wish that I had. It wasn't that I was disgusted, but that I was terrified, paralyzed. I was afraid I wouldn't do it right, that I would spill the pan, or hurt my mother. But more than that, I was afraid of what this meant for our relationship. I wasn't ready for this kind of inversion. I knew my mother wasn't ready for it, either. She didn't ask me to do it, but clearly someone needed to do it.

I don't know how long it took the nurse to come in and help, but it felt like a long time. And I don't blame the nurse: My mother wasn't going to die from lying on that bedpan, and there were probably other patients who needed the nurse for more acute problems. This is very, very far from the worst thing that can happen when there just aren't enough nurses per patient. But the memory is infused with a terrible dark regret that stays with me always.

Nurse labor organizations have chipped away at the fundamental problems in nurses' working conditions, which could help alleviate staffing problems—as came to pass in California. National Nurses United said it has organized nearly five thousand nurses from eight different hospital systems since the pandemic began, more workers than any other single union during this period. Unionization means that nurses can force hospitals to provide adequate staffing and personal protective equipment (like fitted N95s) through contract bargaining. A federal law that would set nationwide minimum nurse staffing ratios has been introduced in Congress, and NNU is lobbying for its passage. But as of now, ratio laws proposed in states besides California have failed to pass and have been actively opposed by the American Nurses Association. So, the very same old problems are still destabilizing our health care system, and Covid-19 has only revealed and deepened them. Nurse labor leaders say that, once again, they are in a moment ripe for revolution—because, once again, conditions are as bad as they ever have been.

The U.S. health care system is wobbling in the wake of Covid-19, as more nurses than ever find that they simply can't bear their working conditions. By now, we know these stories, but they bear repeating: During the pandemic, nurses have been asked to work without proper protection, have been the only witness to death upon death upon death. Some nurses have died themselves as a result of exposures at work. At the beginning of the pandemic, nurses were put on furlough or laid off because, without elective procedures being performed, revenue wasn't flowing into hospitals. Then they were frantically called back to work that, by some accounts, left half of all nurses with posttraumatic stress disorder.

The novel coronavirus pandemic inspired a groundswell of gratitude for nurses and for all health care workers. In 2020, Brooklyn's spring and summer evenings were filled with the sound of applause as we emerged onto our stoops or leaned out our windows to cheer the health care workers fighting Covid-19 in our city's overwhelmed hospitals. Sirens wailed, and the crematorium down the street streamed white smoke day and night. It was comforting to express this gratitude, especially to express it ritualistically as a community, thinking that nurses would hold the line for us no matter what. We sent them pizzas and flowers; we called them our heroes—and we meant it. But this wasn't really what they needed.

In April 2020, Cortney, a registered nurse at Brigham and Women's Hospital in Boston, suddenly found herself alone. Usually, she enjoys working with a large interdisciplinary team of physicians, respiratory and swallow therapists, nursing assistants, and social workers. But there were no patients except Covid-19 patients, and she was the only person entering their rooms. She had been assigned to a Covid step-down unit, tending to patients who were not quite sick enough for the ICU but not well enough for a regular medical floor. And this floor was always full of patients. The physicians performed exams and managed communication mostly from an iPad screen. (Though when a patient needed to be intubated, for example, physicians did have to go in the room.) Therapists also consulted remotely, and housekeeping couldn't enter Covid-19 rooms anymore, either.

What this meant was that Cortney was now solely responsible for her patients. She administered their medications; assessed their mental state, vital signs, and respiratory status; adjusted the care as necessary, consulting with the physicians remotely. She emptied the trash, changed sheets, bathed patients, and delivered their meals. Because family and friends couldn't visit, Cortney was her patients' one and only source of human contact: "We have to provide all the psycho-social support, the emotional support that our patients need," she said. This was especially painful for patients, but also for her. "Everything is falling on us, for every aspect of patient care. I am doing the jobs of five different people. You never stop."

The hospital's policy on who could enter the rooms of patients with Covid-19 was designed to limit the number of people potentially exposed, and there weren't enough masks to go around. Meanwhile, Cortney was reusing PPE, a previously unthinkable practice. She was allowed *one* N95 mask per shift, and then she said all the masks would go through a mysterious new sterilizing process so they could be used again. The fact that nurses were the only ones going into the rooms was a tacit acknowledgment that, when it came down to it, nursing work was the most indispensable patient care that happened in the hospital.

The experience of Covid-19 has changed the way Cortney thinks about her work. As 2022 began, she was about to finish her master's degree, which would allow her to transition to a role in clinical nurse education at the hospital and do less direct patient care. She was always interested in teaching, but the pandemic has accelerated her plans. She is eager to leave the bedside.

Tiffany, a registered nurse who worked at a major academic hospital center in New Orleans, had a similar experience. She also worked as a step-down nurse, and in the summer of 2020, the hospital was full of Covid-19 patients. Tiffany explained that no one went into these patients' rooms except for nurses. "You can't let someone lay in bed and not provide care," she said. "We do still have doctors. They've been doing their assessments from the doorway."

In late 2021, after working five straight days during Hurricane Ida amid the height of the Delta wave of the coronavirus, Tiffany decided she had had enough. It wasn't just those five days. It was also that the hospital had given up fit-testing nurses for N95s, so she wasn't sure she was being protected against the virus and didn't feel her hospital cared if she was. It was that there were never enough nurses for a given shift. It was that certified nursing assistants were quitting because they were being paid twelve dollars an hour, and they could get more than that working retail and not risk their lives.

So, Tiffany quit—as did the majority of the nurses in her unit. She took a lucrative short-term travel nurse contract that sent her to a hospital in the Kansas City area because the money offered a way out. She wanted to take time off to think about how to make a living next. She wasn't sure if she still wanted to be a nurse.

Nurses I spoke to recognized that all the hero talk came from a good place, but they also found it wearying. It indicated that the public didn't really understand the work they did—didn't really understand it as skilled work, not an immutable identity. Nurses don't *owe* us their labor. But of course, we do *need* nurses. (*We* meaning all of us, including nurses themselves.) So the only solution is to treat nurses fairly, as indispensable workers, with appropriate compensation and safe working conditions. As the experience in California shows, when these measures are instituted, many nurses *want* to work at the bedside.

Covid-19 might be a novel virus, but the pandemic played out in ways that showed how the past is not at all past. Who was protected and who was not? Who was expected to sacrifice? These false archetypes persist: Caring is done by indentured girls. It's done by enslaved women. It's done by nuns. By mothers. By witchy old women. At the end of the fifteenth century, in Florence, Italy, these ideas played out in a dramatic way during a syphilis epidemic. The disease, sometimes called the pox, was highly stigmatized because of its conspicuous smelly rash and its association with sex workers. Everyone was eager to blame someone else for it: the British called it the French disease, the French called it the Neapolitan disease, North Africans called it the Spanish disease, and the Turks called it the Christian disease.

At a Florentine pox hospital, the nurses were impoverished young women who were required to be virgins and who were indentured to the hospital for life. The rationale was that, if they were not "saved" by becoming nurses, these young women would otherwise become prostitutes who might then spread the pox. Francesca, an impoverished sixteen-year-old orphan girl from Prato, was exactly the sort of nurse whom the hospital officials loved to recruit. Pox nurses like Francesca administered medications and elaborate remedies like the "wood cure," which involved burning small wood stoves to heat up the wards and make the patients sweat copiously. They did the laundry and the cooking. They emptied chamber pots. It was easy to get injured helping patients move to and fro, washing huge loads of bedding over wood fires, cleaning up vomit and sweat and feces. On Saturdays, these nurses went around town to beg for alms.

The idea of these nurses' purity made other people feel safer, while the nurses themselves were not safe at all. In her book *Forgotten Healers*, historian Sharon T. Strocchia, PhD, describes how these nurses played a "compensatory role" within the community's anxieties over contagion, health, and morality: "Pox nurses helped purify the city as moral agents who offset the effects of sexual vice." They were symbols. In a way, they were sacrifices.

Later, when the meaning of our own pandemic fractured around arguments over what safety and care we owed one another, with nurses working in the fallout of wave after wave, I thought of those virgin pox nurses in fifteenth-century Florence, how they served as counterweights to panic, how their work was essential, but how their individual lives were treated as disposable.

But in the present day, forcing people to work in terrible conditions can backfire. Those who can will start to refuse, to quit, to strike. Right now, no one—not hospitals and not nurses and not nurse labor organizations—thinks hospital nurse staffing is functioning well. They just disagree about the locus of the blame. One recent target of hospital ire has been travel nurses like Tiffany. Hospitals often must hire travel nurses when they don't have enough staff nurses to operate. Travel nurses are contract workers who fill vacancies for weeks or months and are often paid about twice what staff nurses are. Part of this deal, though, is that they don't have job security, must be willing to leave home and family to work, and don't get benefits like health insurance and retirement plans. In recent years, travel nursing has boomed, a symptom of an unstable system. For Tiffany, as for many nurses, travel nursing wasn't something she particularly wanted to do; she felt pushed to do it—as in *You can treat me poorly or pay me poorly, but not both.* It's not a sustainable solution, but who can blame nurses for turning the tables and charging what the market will bear? The American Hospital Association (AHA) has demanded a congressional investigation into travel nursing's high wages. It does not object to a profit-driven health care model in general, only to nurses using the market to their advantage.

The system is wobbling, but the system has always wobbled. No one knows what will come next. Brogan of the NNU is loath to predict the future. "I've seen more confidence within the nursing profession. More giving the finger, basically. *No, I'm not doing this anymore. Screw you.* But on the other hand, I've seen more moves by the hospital industry to replace us: Splitting up what nurses have done historically into smaller bits. Fragmented, lesser paid, lesser trained. So, it's a matter of who's going to win that fight, I think."

The American Hospital Association, which represents about five thousand hospitals and health care systems, disputes just about all this. It argues that the staffing issues are occurring because of the toll the pandemic has taken—essentially, an act of God—and that, as a result, labor costs have risen at an unsustainable clip. "Hospitals also have incurred significant costs in recruiting and retaining staff, which have included overtime pay, bonus pay and other incentives," the group stated in a 2022 workforce brief.

The brief acknowledged that burnout was a factor and suggested wellness services to prevent it—providing nurses with therapists, mindfulness practices, and gym memberships. I recently heard a hospital's corporate nursing officer interviewed on NPR, suggesting that nurses just really need a vacation. These amenities may be helpful for some people, but researchers investigating nurse burnout—now often called moral injury—found that it is highly correlated with stressful work environments and inadequate staffing. A vacation or a yoga class can't solve those larger issues.

Meanwhile, hospital administrator pay has continued to rise in recent years. The CEO of Hospital Corporation of America made over thirty million dollars in 2020. Even nonprofit hospital systems pay CEOs and administrators astronomic salaries. Unlike the correlation between nurse staffing and patient outcomes, researchers have found no correlation between hospital CEO pay and hospital mortality, readmission rates, or value to the community. This is a jarring asymmetry that raises larger questions: What is the purpose of a hospital? And should a hospital's budget reflect its purpose?

But there is a sense that this broken moment might present a new way forward, a great rebalancing. Perhaps this could be a moment of nursing power: The gratitude we in the public feel for nurses could be harnessed to more active support for nursing work. And nurses themselves, after so many years of being pushed to their limits, might be more willing to engage in collective action. In some places, this is happening. After complaints about unsafe working conditions were ignored, nurses at Saint Vincent Hospital in Worcester, Massachusetts, recently waged a strike for nearly a year. Their primary demand was increased nurse staffing, and they won it. In September 2022, fifteen thousand Minnesota nurses walked off the job for three days to demand higher levels of staffing, a dispute that is ongoing. And in January 2023, more than seven thousand New York City nurses went on strike for three days and won increased staffing.

In 2021, Erin, an ICU nurse who had previously worked at UCLA Health, took a travel contract to work at Mount Sinai in Manhattan, when she and her husband moved there. Erin was shocked at much of what she saw at Mount Sinai: The contrast between California, with its nurse-to-patient ratio law, and New York, which doesn't have one, was stark. She said some ICU nurses were taking care of four patients, double the recommended number, or working twenty-four-hour shifts. The experience completely changed the way Erin thought about nursing unions.

"When I moved to L.A., I was taken off guard by the union aspect of nursing," she said. "I didn't join [the union] immediately. I felt weird about it. I didn't have that much sympathy. When I first got to UCLA, we went on strike for forty-eight hours. But I actually went to work. I was one of two nurses that went to work on my unit. And I never told anyone that I worked with, because it was not kosher. But personally, I felt like I was abandoning my patients if I went on strike."

While Erin was at Mount Sinai, nurses were holding protests outside the hospital, with the support of the New York State Nurses Association, trying to call attention to the dire staffing conditions inside the hospital. Mount Sinai responded by saying that the hospital valued and fought for its nurses and that the nurse staffing crisis was a nationwide problem, not specific to Mount Sinai. But Erin knew this wasn't exactly true—at UCLA, even at the height of Covid-19, they were almost never short-staffed because the state law prohibited it.

"My perspective is now a little bit different," she said. "At a place like Mount Sinai, nurses are asking for very simple things. They're not even asking for more money. They're just asking for more staffing and for blocking beds, things like that," she says, referring to the practice of limiting the number of patients that can be admitted to a floor based on nurse staffing. "And they're not being listened to. I think it's easy, when you're in administration, to be really removed and think you can just keep putting a Band-Aid on it. Now I think when nurses take action, they're very powerful."

When nurses say they are striking for patient safety, it might sound like just another slogan, but the available evidence shows that it is true that the devaluing of nursing is the devaluing of human lives. It means that someone in charge has tallied up the expenses and decided to make cuts they know will result in worse health for patients. When nurses make this case to the public, it is a powerful message. It is no wonder so much effort has been expended to keep them quiet.

CHAPTER 10

POWER

Taking Charge: What We All Gain When
Good Nurses Govern

New York State assemblywoman Phara Souffrant Forrest, BSN, RN, was in an Albany legislative session in 2022, hammering out the state budget for the following year. A proposal to fund syphilis screening for pregnant women in the third trimester came up for debate. Several legislators wondered out loud why this would be necessary—did people even *get* syphilis anymore? But Forrest knew exactly how urgent syphilis screening was, because in her work as a maternal and child health nurse, she'd seen many pregnant women with the disease, which, if untreated, can be passed to the baby during delivery. And she knew *why* it was happening in her district in Brooklyn, too.

"You still have the issue of a male-dominated culture," she said. "And we're not having proper economic justice for Black women. One in four women will face eviction. So, trust me, they are hanging on to that man for dear life. If he says he wants to have sex without a condom? Guess who ends up in the third trimester with chlamydia, gonorrhea, HIV, syphilis?"

As a nurse in obstetrics and gynecology at Brooklyn's Kings County Medical Center and in maternal health home nursing, Forrest saw this dynamic at work. She pointed out that when women's very survival and the survival of their children depend on the money brought in by a male partner, the women don't always have a choice to defend their bodies. And so, she argued to her fellow lawmakers, yes, it's worth spending the money to screen for syphilis. This was a context most of her fellow lawmakers did not have.

Forrest is charismatic, animated, and funny. She speaks with the authority of a nurse, which she has found to be effective in the legislature, even across party lines. After she spoke up about syphilis, she said, a Republican lawmaker with whom she didn't usually have much in common came over to thank her.

When voting for leaders, Americans seem to consider certain professions a plus. If a political hopeful is an entrepreneur or a businessperson, this is touted as evidence of a certain kind of common sense. Lawyers might have a useful knowledge of the law and the court system. But what about what nurses know?

It is one thing to understand in theory that our health care system is broken and that something ought to be done about it and an entirely different thing to have your hands in the leaky dam of that broken health care system every day. In her nursing career in St. Louis, Congresswoman Cori Bush, RN, saw what happened to patients with diabetes who couldn't afford the three hundred dollars a month for their insulin. They rationed it; they skipped it. As a result, some lost limbs; some fell into comas and died. As an individual nurse, she could do next to nothing to solve this problem: in the United States, insulin is more expensive than it is in other countries. But now, as a member of Congress who has that nursing knowledge, she is working on legislation that could put a thirty-five-dollar monthly cap on insulin costs for patients. (The Inflation Reduction Act of 2022 included the $35 cap for Medicare patients, but Republicans blocked efforts to extend that cap to all.) She ran for Congress, Bush said, to make manifest the fact that health care is a human right. She lost in 2016 and 2018 before winning by 60 percentage points in 2020, the Year of the Nurse.

Bush and Forrest are two of a growing number of nurses who, driven by systemic problems they've seen in their work, are running for, and often winning, political office. They are taking the lead on expanding access to health care and writing policy focusing on social determinants of health—like housing, schools, and air and water quality. These nurses see their political work as a direct extension of their nursing careers.

There are now two nurses in Congress, Representative Bush, and Rep. Lauren Underwood. Pennsylvania state house representative Tarik S. Khan is a nurse practitioner; New York City councilwoman Mercedes Narcisse is a nurse, as is Minnesota state senator Erin Murphy and two newly elected Wisconsin assemblypersons. It feels like a movement, one that has been a long time coming, one that might be further propelled by nurses' increased visibility during the Covid-19 pandemic. According to a yearly Gallup poll, for twenty years running, the public has ranked nursing as the most ethical and honest profession. That trust is a kind of power—but only if it is used, and used to a purpose. Maybe this is what it looks like to take that famous public trust and leverage it to make change. Maybe this is what it looks like to nurse the system.

Nursing has a method for making personalized care plans for patients, and several nurses in politics told me that the method works with policy, too. It involves a series of steps: assess, plan, implement, and evaluate (often referred to as APIE). And if the desired outcome isn't reached, you loop back around to assess again and make a different plan.

It works like this: When a patient is being discharged, a nurse first *assesses* the situation: say the patient is a premature baby who still needs to gain weight, and the mom is struggling with pumping and mental health issues. The nurse then *plans*: for example, a home health nurse will go to the home every other day to weigh the baby and check in with the mom on feeding. At that point, the nurse *intervenes*, providing the planned care. Then the nurse *evaluates*: Is the baby gaining weight? Is the mom managing and getting help? If the answer is yes, the care plan has worked. If no, the nurse returns to the first step, reassesses, and tries something different.

Forrest finds it frustrating to see policy work utterly fail in meeting this standard for efficacy. Legislatures put programs into practice but rarely go back and evaluate if those programs have been successful. If nurses worked the way legislators do, she said, they'd lose their licenses. "Nurses are the ultimate project managers. As a nurse, I have to have a rationale for *everything*. I have a rationale for *bedsheets*. Why do we make beds the way we do? Because we don't want to have the patient with bed sores and marks on their skin. So, you're telling me you have a program for the Department of Health. Where is the data?"

Nursing is political simply because health and caring are deeply linked to how a nation chooses to treat its citizens. And when nurses use their knowledge to fight for positive change on a grand scale, they are doing so within a long tradition of nurses in political action.

Some nurses have always been radical, though certainly not all: In 1907, the Nurses Associated Alumnae (precursor to the American Nurses Association) voted resoundingly against supporting the cause of women's suffrage. In 1908, veteran nurse Lavinia L. Dock, RN— the same Lavinia Dock who cowrote *A History of Nursing*—wrote a letter to the editor at *The American Journal of Nursing*, to express her shock and humiliation that this group of nurses did not think that they themselves should have the right and the duty to vote. She went on to argue passionately that what nurses know, what nurses were interested in, were fundamentally social issues that had to be addressed on a large scale, politically. "Take the present question of the underfed school children in New York. How many of them will have tuberculosis? If mothers and nurses had votes there might be school lunches for all those children." (A beautiful argument, though it would turn out to be overly optimistic.)

This is the same argument Forrest used to advocate for syphilis testing: The disease is never *just* the disease. Health problems are often caused by larger societal problems, and nurses are uniquely situated to understand and address this--but they must be willing to act politically to do so. The ANA resisted supporting women's suffrage out of a sense of conservatism, a reluctance to cause offense, and a desire to maintain the status quo. In a very direct echo, in 2020, the ANA failed to endorse a candidate for president for the first time since 1988, citing their concern that choosing a side would be too divisive.

Lavinia Dock was born into a well-to-do Pennsylvania family in 1858, one of five sisters, none of whom ever married. After graduating from the Bellevue Hospital School of Nursing, she went to Florida to care for patients during an outbreak of yellow fever, working alongside Jane Delano, who would later lead the Red Cross. Dock then went to Johnstown, Pennsylvania, to help flood victims, working with Clara Barton, founder of the Red Cross. In the meantime, she wrote *Materia Medica for Nurses*, the first nurse handbook on medications, which eventually sold one hundred thousand copies and was used in nursing schools all over the country.

But it was in 1896, when she was thirty-eight, that she later said she learned to think. This was when she moved to the Henry Street

Settlement to work with Lillian Wald and started engaging in political action. She became an activist in the labor and women's suffrage movements, which she saw as consistent with her efforts to move nursing toward scientific professionalism and autonomy.

The same year Dock moved to Henry Street, she was arrested for attempting to vote in New York City. Over the next decades, she dedicated herself to women's suffrage: She joined the National Woman's Party (NWP), the most radical and militant wing of the suffrage movement. With a group of other suffragists, she walked for about three weeks from New York City to Washington, DC, to join a women's protest in which the marchers were kicked, tripped, grabbed, and shoved by jeering men. In 1917, while picketing outside the White House, she was arrested again. The *Evening News* in Dock's hometown of Harrisburg, Pennsylvania, reported it this way: "Miss Dock, a tiny woman of 60 years, made a determined effort against the six-foot policeman to retain the possession of her banner."

This moment marked a turning point in how severely suffragists were punished. Dock was sentenced to thirty days in Occoquan Workhouse, in Virginia, a brutal prison where suffragists were shoved and beaten, stripped naked by guards, chained to the bars, and force-fed raw eggs. And yet, Dock picketed at the White House again, and was again arrested and sent back to Occoquan, and this time she sustained a severe leg injury from a guard. It was a violent experience, though she later made light of it, writing, "It was a great joy to do a little guerilla war in that cause, and I believe that going to jail gave me a purer feeling of unalloyed content than I ever had in any of my other work."

Dock's actions rebutted a common, milquetoast idea that nurses should somehow be "above" politics, outside the fray. In a 1913 article in *The American Journal of Nursing*, she wrote, "No nurse should be opposed to enfranchisement for women. . . . If we are exclusive and shut our minds to all except 'professional' subjects, we shall become one-sided specialists and in time lose our usefulness."

The legacy of this idea—that political action *is* nursing—is still controversial among nurses, who sometimes fear retaliation from their institutions for speaking freely or who perhaps have been socialized not to speak up. But as the Covid-19 pandemic put both nurses and public health policy at center stage, the inherent political nature of nursing is becoming more visible, less avoidable: recall the nurses in masks who silently confronted the anti-mask protesters in Arizona in 2020. Some nurses feel they now *must* take what they know to a wider audience, where it can have more of an impact. In fact, this played out in one of 2021's most hotly contested elections.

Being at the bedside has two meanings, and India Walton, ASN, RN, who became a progressive star when she ran for mayor of Buffalo in 2021, has lived both. Walton's first son, who has sickle cell anemia, was born when she was just fourteen. Walton lived in a group home for young mothers, worked, and got her GED. Then, when she was nineteen years old, her twin sons were born at twenty-four weeks' gestation. The boys spent six months in the NICU. Walton had experienced more of American health care before she was twenty than many people do their whole lives. She felt that much of the care she and her sons received had been cold and unempathetic because she was a young, poor, Black mother. This is what made her decide to become a nurse: so that she could improve on that care. And it crystalized her conviction that the truest role of a nurse is advocate.

Twenty years later, I met Walton in downtown Buffalo on a cold, blustery November day a few weeks after the mayoral election. She had a calm directness about her, and her smile was infectious. She has enviable posture that maybe brings her to five feet; that day, she wore a black head wrap with jeans and a black-and-red-checked flannel shirt.

When Walton ran for mayor of Buffalo, she became a political celebrity practically overnight–specifically, the night she won the Democratic primary in a stunning upset. She hadn't expected that level of fame, and she found it disconcerting. But her career as a nurse had given her a certain comfort with discomfort. For many years, she worked at the NICU at the John R. Oishei Children's Hospital of Buffalo, where her own sons were cared for. With the insight of a mother with a critically ill child, Walton had a visceral understanding that nothing about the NICU was normal or routine.

"I'm used to popping an IV into a baby's scalp because it's easy to do, and sometimes I might have to shave their head. But before I do that, I'm thinking about what this mother is going to see, what this father's going to see, what these siblings are going to see, when they get there. It only takes two minutes, even if you had to do it emergently, to just give them a call and say, 'Hey, I just want you to know we had to start a new IV.'"

Walton left the NICU to become a school nurse in Buffalo Public Schools. There, she noticed that most of the kids who ended up in her office didn't have a simple physical ailment that she could treat– a stomach bug, a scrape from a playground fall, strep throat. Instead, it was more like this: There was the little girl who had lice. Walton told her mom that if she shampooed the girl's hair with delousing shampoo that evening, she could come back to school the next day. The mother said this would be impossible. She didn't get paid until Friday, so she couldn't buy the shampoo until then. So, the girl wouldn't be back until Monday. Walton realized that this girl was going to miss three days of school unnecessarily. As a nurse, she wanted to help people and solve problems, but this problem wasn't really about the lice.

Walton has given this a lot of thought. "We have education advocates saying teachers aren't doing enough. We have teachers saying that parents aren't doing enough. Then you have the little school nurse over in the corner, like, 'Y'all are all wrong.' The problem in our school system is concentrated poverty, disadvantage, community violence. . . . We send children who are housing-insecure, hungry, and tired to a school building. We throw them in the classroom with thirty-two other kids, one teacher, and then we give them Pop-Tarts and brownies for breakfast. Then we feed them an overprocessed lunch while we deny them art and music—and we wonder why they're bouncing off the walls. A political science degree is not going to help you figure that out."

So, she took her nursing insight and ran for mayor as a Democratic Socialist. She ran against the four-term incumbent, Democrat Byron Brown, whom Walton characterizes as arrogant at best and a right-winger in centrist Democrat's clothing at worst. Brown wouldn't debate her; he barely even campaigned. Then, in the primary, she beat him.

The Buffalo mayoral race is not normally big national news, but in heavily Democratic cities, winning the Democratic primary is akin to winning the mayor's race altogether. The upset was dramatic. It was David versus Goliath; it was a shot across the bow of the Democratic establishment of New York State. *The New Yorker* ran a profile of Walton, and so did *The Nation*. MSNBC's Chris Hayes interviewed her on his podcast. *Washington Monthly* magazine called her "the AOC of Lake Erie." The *New York Post* sounded slightly hysterical: "Socialist India Walton Wins Mayoral Primary in Buffalo Shocker."

But Byron Brown was not going quietly. He launched a full-scale write-in campaign instead: "Write down Byron Brown." Meanwhile, New York State governor Kathy Hochul declined to endorse Walton, as did many other prominent New York Democrats, even though party leaders almost always endorse the winners of primary elections. Brown has deep roots in the Democratic Party in the state and is an ally of former governor Andrew Cuomo. Walton kept campaigning hard. She ran with slogans that made the point that social issues were also health issues: "Housing is health care," "Infrastructure is health care," "Immigration is health care."

On November 2, 2021, Walton lost to Brown's write-in campaign in the general election. But her nursing-informed policy ideas have changed the conversation in Buffalo and nationwide. Walton's leadership career isn't over—but even if she never runs for office again, she showed, against all odds, that established political machines aren't invincible. And now other nurses are reimagining what is possible.

One of them is Tarik S. Khan, PhD, CRNP, a Democrat from Philadelphia. In 2022, Khan ran against an entrenched incumbent for a state house of representatives seat and prevailed in an underdog win. He had decided to run for office when, in 2021, he got the idea to distribute unused doses of the Covid-19 vaccine to homebound seniors. The health center where he works often had extra doses at the end of the day, and they had to be used within a matter of hours. Meanwhile, many low-income or disabled seniors in the community were both the most vulnerable to the infection and the least likely to be able to come get the vaccine. Khan wanted to match surplus to need, but getting the go-ahead was a bureaucratic nightmare. The clock was running out on these doses; he was texting and calling and emailing to get approval and, all of a sudden, he thought, "Why is this so hard? Shouldn't bureaucracy work *for* people and not against them?"

He finally got the approvals he needed, and ever since, he has spent his off-hours driving around Philadelphia giving out vaccines. But it was obvious to him that the status quo wasn't working in multiple ways: he saw it in the lives of his patients, many of whom had multiple jobs and were barely surviving.

Even before running for state office, Khan was politically active, and he has always seen that work as part of nursing practice. He is outspokenly progressive but also a pragmatist. He resists characterizing all nursing issues–things like union protections, access to health care, or being able to transfer a Pennsylvania nursing license to another state–as partisan: "You can't look at a licensing question and say this is a Republican or Democratic issue," he said. In 2020, he was the president of the Pennsylvania State Nurses Association, the state branch of the American Nurses Association. He felt he was able to be effective at the ANA when it came to licensing issues and the like, and he was proud of this. But the refusal of the ANA to endorse a candidate in the 2020 election deeply rankled him.

Khan does not see any advantage to nurses staying politically neutral. The ANA's silence on the matter seemed to offend his conviction that nurses put common sense above all else. His mom is a nurse, too. "When I think about her and her nurse friends, the way they dealt with stuff, it was no bullshit: problem-focused, help the patient get what they need." So, in 2021–amid the unchecked coronavirus pandemic, the empty neutrality, the red tape–he looked around and concluded that his community was not getting what it needed, and he didn't see leaders rising to the occasion. As nurses often do, he decided to do something himself.

His policy goals are informed by his patients and include Medicare for All, an increase in the minimum wage, and the creation of infrastructure to mitigate climate change's impacts on working-class neighborhoods. The current system is not working for the people he cares for: "They're working seventy hours a week and barely making it. And there's no end in sight. I've seen that as a nurse. So, when I hear these talking points, like, 'If people just work hard' or 'They just have to be resourceful, and they're going to be fine.' Actually, they are doing all those things, and they're *not fine*."

For Khan, these issues represent the forces entwined in people's lives that can make health and happiness possible or impossible. His hope is that nurses' increased visibility during the Covid-19 pandemic will lead to more good nurses in political power, where they can put their pragmatic, people-centered expertise to work. "If we expect to have better leadership, we need nurses in positions of power. Nurses are *overqualified*. We're educators, we're clinicians, we're scientists, we're laborers. We have so much perspective that's needed."

New York State assemblywoman Forrest has a touchstone for everything she does, one that resonates both in nursing and in policy work: *Fanm se poto mitan*. It's a Haitian saying that means, roughly, "Women are the central pillar." Without them, everything falls down. Forrest had an awakening to its truth while working in obstetrics and gynecology at Kings County Hospital Center in Brooklyn. "When you address the needs of women, you can see it's actually child care; it's education; it's the workforce. It's environmental justice," she said. Pregnant people build the future in their own bodies. "So, you're shaping the future when you focus on women's health."

In *her* body, Forrest holds the stories of the people she has cared for. She carries them with her into the halls of Albany, and that knowledge shapes everything she does. She noticed, for instance, that she was seeing more cervical cancer in her community. The cancer was being caught too late, because people weren't getting screened, and they hadn't gotten the HPV vaccine, which prevents cervical cancer. Forrest was looking at the data, trying to figure out the cause of the rise in rates, when she realized that many of those people were currently or formerly incarcerated and that the prisons were not providing routine gynecological care. So, she wrote a bill that would mandate that incarcerated people have access to yearly preventative gynecological care in prison; it has yet to come to a vote, but Forrest will keep introducing it until it does.

When we spoke, she was also working on a bill that would

mandate home health aides be paid at least 150 percent of the hourly state minimum wage, which would bring them to about $22 an hour. That would mean that the people who do the most intimate, difficult nursing care for people in their homes would at least get paid more than they would as cooks at McDonald's. Right now, there's a serious shortage of home care workers, not because they don't exist, but because they can earn more elsewhere, doing less difficult, less dangerous work. Unfortunately, the compromise bill that ultimately passed increased home health workers' wages by only one to two dollars over the minimum wage in 2022, with an additional dollar to be added in 2023.

Forrest points out that when people hear about low wages for home health aides, they think, "Woe is *them*," she said. "It should be 'Woe is *us*.' If I don't pay health care workers fairly today, where will that leave me tomorrow? What if my mom needs care? And then, what about my kid? We need universal child care. Nurses are very clear on certain things."

In her campaign materials, Forrest is pictured in scrubs, with a stethoscope around her neck. Her arms are crossed, and she's smiling gently at the camera, her hair in loose curls. She projects care and competence, a clear leveraging of that public trust afforded nurses. But next time, she wants to present a sharper, tougher image of herself, as a nurse. She wants people to understand that nurses don't *just* care but are *effective*—that there's nothing soft about what she brings to the job.

"The other side of nurses is that we don't play," she said. "I negotiate. I crunch the numbers. I do the policy, read between the lines, understand, and digest. Right? And then, I deliver."

LOVE IN ACTION

Nursing is love in action.

—LILLIAN WALD

There is nothing more urgent than understanding the potential power of nursing right now. In the reporting of this book, I spoke to nurses who practice in thoughtful, innovative ways that respond to the innate right of every person and community to be valued and cared for. At a time of discord in the United States, amid the rise of antidemocratic forces and health care system breakdown, I was spending my days talking to people who had dedicated their lives to helping people—by providing support for those with diabetes; by helping the dying do so peacefully and surrounded by love; by making reproductive care accessible; by changing the way those with substance use disorder are treated; by protecting farmworkers from heatstroke; and by passing policy to improve people's lives. The work they do is quieter than the cacophony, but it is powerful, and it is old. If there is a human instinct to tear apart, to hurt and destroy, there is also a human instinct to mend, to care, to reach out. These nurses helped me believe that caring and partnership are smarter and more potent than domination and violence.

These nurses represent the present and the future of the oldest nursing traditions, which call us to remember that caring for one another is what makes us human—*and* that we must all work at that every day. We can build a better world, one in which the most humane values of nursing can be realized.

I started working on this book right before the pandemic descended. When it did, like everyone else who wasn't essential, I was stuck at home conducting interviews over Zoom and doing a lot of reading. The second I was vaccinated, I wanted to start interviewing people in person. Writing a book about the healing power of human relationships is much harder when you can't see people.

When Marcella Rose Ryan LeBeau, RN, agreed to meet with me, I flew out to South Dakota to interview her. LeBeau, who was also known by her Lakota name, "Wígmuŋke Wašté Wín," or "Pretty Rainbow Woman," had nursed during World War II. She was 101 years old and had been a nurse her whole life, a great swath of the twentieth and twenty-first centuries. I wanted to ask her how nursing had changed in all that time. I wanted to hear about nursing from a Native American perspective. But what I wasn't prepared for was that LeBeau would show me, more than anyone else, how *vast* nursing can be. Her scope of practice was *life*: anything that affected the well-being of her community was within the purview of her nursing. And her work was grounded in how well she knew and loved her neighbors. She knew their histories and their families and the conditions they lived in. She *was* them. She knew how to provide nursing care, and she understood the many causes of health and illness. She put those ways of knowing together, and the result was the deepest kind of wisdom. Not placid wisdom: there was rage and sorrow in her wisdom, and action, and the hard kind of hope that is grounded in knowing exactly how far there is to go.

LeBeau graduated from nursing school as World War II raged and the nurse shortage was all over the news. She volunteered for the Army Nurse Corps. (No one seems to have noticed she wasn't white, though she was open about being Lakota.) She was stationed in the United Kingdom, France, and Belgium; she nursed casualties of D-day and the Battle of the Bulge—a blur of blood transfusions and penicillin injections and prepping soldiers for emergency surgery. She worked in a surgical unit in a thousand-bed field hospital under heavy bombardment by Luftwaffe buzz bombs, whose percussive assault often came every few minutes. Her hospital unit followed the Allied forces marching from the beaches of Normandy to liberate Europe. She remembers one night that sounded like a scene from *Casablanca*: Her unit was camped in a French cow pasture. A local Frenchwoman came out and set up long tables, set with her best tablecloths and silverware, and cooked big pots of food for them. Before the woman served the food, she stood and sang "La Marseillaise," the French national anthem, with tears running down her face. LeBeau experienced all this, and then she went home to nurse her community, the Lakota Oyate.

On a sunny, hot June day in 2021, I drove from Pierre, the capital of South Dakota, to LeBeau's bright-pink stone home in Eagle Butte, part of the sovereign Lakota Nation of the Cheyenne River Sioux Tribe. She lived alone, but one daughter resided in the house next door. LeBeau greeted me in her living room, where photos of her children and grandchildren grinned from every surface. Her silvery hair was twisted up, and she was wearing a neat black suit with a sequined flower on her lapel. She was very beautiful and still looked much like she did in a photo of her as a twentysomething army nurse, wearing a dark suit-jacketed uniform and jaunty cap, lipsticked and smiling.

After the war, LeBeau got married and had eight children. She worked as a nurse at the Indian Health Service hospital in Eagle Butte, where she stayed for over thirty years. It was a small hospital, and she did every kind of nursing: surgical, emergency, obstetrics-gynecology, intensive care. At least once, she delivered a baby on a tiny airplane while en route to a bigger hospital. ("It was about half-way through the flight; she said the baby was coming. So, I said, 'Go right ahead.'") The baby was named Angel Marcella, because she was born close to heaven and delivered by Marcella LeBeau. LeBeau loved being useful to her community. "I think there's great satisfaction in being able to help other people," she said.

We chatted in her house for a while, but she was recently vaccinated and wanted to take a drive. So, we got in my rental car and went cruising through the town. Main Street in Eagle Butte is a wide stretch of about four blocks lined with low-slung wooden and brick buildings. We drove slowly past a steak house, the tiny headquarters of the *West River Eagle* newspaper, the post office, and the tribal government building. LeBeau sat in the passenger seat pointing out landmarks. She knew who lived in every house, and she had three generations' worth of gossip about them. It soon became clear to me that I wasn't getting a tour of the town. I was getting a tour of how LeBeau's nursing perspective worked, and how it was grounded in this place, with these people.

"This is the tribal building," she said, pointing out a wide wooden building where the Tribal Council works. She explained to me how it and all the public buildings on the reservation had come to prohibit smoking.

When she was a Tribal Council member in the 1990s, she made herself a spreadsheet, one row at the top for the names of her fellow council members and a column beneath each name. Every time someone lit up a cigarette, a little check would go below their name, along with the time. LeBeau conspicuously logged everyone's smoking habits, gathering the data to prove that smoking was a problem. "It didn't make me very popular," she said. But she was convinced it was necessary for the tribe's health. She was particularly worried about the effects of second- and thirdhand smoke on the tribe's children and elders. She put up giant posters of autopsied diseased lungs in the Tribal Council office and in tribal buildings all over town. After people complained that the posters were too upsetting, not to mention unappetizing, she took them down but started putting smoking cessation flyers and pamphlets in the other council members' mailboxes. Her brother sent her a gas mask as a joke, and she hung it prominently on the wall behind her desk.

The smoke-free resolution was voted down more times than she could remember, over the course of nearly two decades, but she never stopped proposing it. Finally, in 2015, it passed, and the Cheyenne River Sioux Reservation was the first Native nation in South Dakota to ban smoking in public spaces.

We drove out to the edge of the town, to the new Indian Health Service hospital. It has clever cultural design details and a special circular space where people can burn sage and not set off the fire alarm. But LeBeau was not impressed. "Up ahead is the twenty-five-million-dollar, state-of-the-art hospital," she said acidly. "And it has eight beds—which to me is almost criminal. We had a thirty-bed hospital in the past, at the old hospital. It's all swept away now. We had surgery, OB, ICU, nursery, emergency room. Now they have eight beds." LeBeau viewed this insufficient eight-bed hospital in the context of the long and ongoing theft from her community: theft of the larger hospital; theft of children, land, and culture. Theft that had led to the suffering and ill health of her neighbors.

The nearest hospital after this one is ninety miles away. This means that most people from the community who need hospitalization must be transferred. It means that their loved ones—if they don't have reliable transportation or work long hours—have difficulty visiting them or, in some cases, can't visit them at all. Transferring patients is expensive and can be less effective. People recover better when their loved ones can be with them.

LeBeau said that when she worked at the Indian Health Service hospital, it was staffed mainly with nurses from the community and with physicians from elsewhere who worked there for a couple of years to get their student loans forgiven. This dynamic brought some challenges, but LeBeau had mostly fond memories of her decades there. The IHS hospital provided standard "Western" medical care. Much of the traditional knowledge about healing plants and herbs had died with her grandmother's generation. Still, traces of it remained: sometimes she'd find a particular root tucked under a patient's pillow, a plant Lakota people believe has antiseptic effects.

When LeBeau was a small child, her mother, Florence Four Bear Ryan, got very sick with a tumor. LeBeau remembered bringing her mother a glass of water when she was in the hospital and how good it felt to provide that small, necessary thing. After the physicians said there was nothing they could do for her, Florence went home to the family's small log house with a big garden, by the Owl River in Promise, South Dakota. There, LeBeau's maternal grandmother, Louise Bear Face Four Bear, nursed her daughter until she died. LeBeau remembered her grandmother's traditional knowledge of medicinal herbs and roots. "My grandmother had learning far beyond education," LeBeau said. "She was full of wisdom."

After LeBeau's mother and grandmother died, LeBeau's father sent all five of his children to an Indian boarding school. The facility was one of hundreds of residential "schools" where the Canadian and American governments, often contracting with the Catholic Church, forcibly kept Native and Indigenous children away from their families, forbade them from speaking their native language or engaging in their culture's traditions, and abused them in every way imaginable. It was part of an attempt to erase Native cultures forever, and Canada has acknowledged it as a cultural genocide. The schools' ethos was "Kill the Indian, save the man." In the United States, a governmental policy in 1869 mandated that Native children be placed in one of these 350 schools. By the middle of the twentieth century, hundreds of thousands of Native children had passed through one of these schools.

LeBeau remembered all of it: The staff routinely beat the children and forced them to work in the laundry or kitchen most of the day, leaving little time for learning. Her brothers quickly learned to fight to avoid being raped. Children often tried to run away. LeBeau remembered one little boy who froze to death trying to get home to his family. Other runaways were recaptured and whipped.

The LeBeau children spoke both English and Lakota. In the school, Lakota was forbidden, and LeBeau saw what happened to children who couldn't speak English. She remembers one of her friends in particular. "She was ten years old, and they took her by her hair and pulled her face up and down, like that," she said, showing me, "to say yes. And then they slapped her face back and forth for no. That was how she learned how to say yes and no."

LeBeau's father, who was white, was allowed to visit her at school occasionally, and she and her siblings begged him to understand what was happening there. "My father was a very kind man," LeBeau said, remembering him as an attentive parent. "He always said, 'Get a good education. No one can take that away from you. Mind your teachers.'" He thought that he was ensuring a good education by sending his children to the boarding school, but eventually, he pulled them all out—perhaps he was able to do so because he was a white man—and sent them to the public high school in a nearby town. There, the siblings got a good education that included Lakota crafts like beading and embroidery.

Almost everyone of a certain age in LeBeau's community spent time at one of these boarding schools. And LeBeau saw how the violence visited on her friends and neighbors as children metastasized as they grew up and had families of their own. She saw increasing health problems from alcohol abuse and from child abuse perpetrated by people who had themselves been abused in the boarding schools. "So, we tried to address that problem. We had workshops and awareness programs. But I was devastated to know that what happened to the children carried on into their adult lives that way."

LeBeau and I kept driving. We passed another shiny, new building. "This is the jail, on the left," she said. "It was a seven- or eight-million-dollar jail. I was on Council when they dedicated it. And I told the lady that it's too bad they can't put this into education. Instead of a jail." The jail has more than eight beds.

We passed modest homes, some in good condition but others not, reflecting the economic struggle of people on this reservation in one of the poorest counties in the country. "We have meth here, like Noem said," LeBeau said, referring to South Dakota governor Kristi Noem's infamous and inexplicable public health campaign featuring the tagline "Meth: We're on it." We passed a larger building, and LeBeau pointed it out. "Here is where we keep some artifacts, like the Ghost Shirt. We have it stored here." The Ghost Shirt is a garment with deep religious significance that was worn by a Lakota person at the 1890 Massacre at Wounded Knee. After the killings, the shirt was stripped from the dead person wearing it and sold as a curiosity to the municipal museum in Glasgow, Scotland. LeBeau, along with several partners, successfully lobbied for years for the return of the stolen shirt, which is still stained with Lakota blood.

As we drove through this small town under a huge sky, mountains rising in the distance, LeBeau was helping me understand that her nursing was a way of seeing her neighbors' pain—which was also her pain—and skillfully responding to it. Her nursing included advocacy for justice because she believed that, without justice, her tribe couldn't be healthy. When LeBeau saw alcoholism, diabetes, and suicide, she knew that those health problems were dark tendrils of the past, manifestations of all that had been taken and continues to be taken from her people. She felt a "pervasive sense of sadness as a result of unresolved grief" on her reservation, and she was compelled to nurse that sadness.

"Take a swing down there," LeBeau said, directing me. We drove by the youth center, with its lush community garden. She told me she is concerned about the mental health of the young people who live here, and she told me about a spate of suicides. "I'm on the Wisdom Keepers board," she said, referring to an advisory board of Lakota elders in the community. "I made a suggestion to the tribe that they should inform the students at the school on depression and anxiety and two-spirited people." *Two-spirited people*—she was using the Lakota cultural term for gender fluid or nonbinary people. "Because few people know. They give two-spirited people a bad time because they don't understand. But in the past, they were valued in our society."

Later, I looked at the obituaries in Eagle Butte's newspaper, the *West River Eagle*. There were: Darci Rae Laurenz, age thirty-three, a mother of three small children; LaToya LaPointe, age thirty-five, a mother of four small children; Nancy Little Shield, thirty-eight; Andrew Little Shield, forty-eight; Melissa Mae Wimberly, age thirty-four; Alan D. Dupris, twenty-eight. These deaths were not from Covid-19—at the time these people passed away, there was only one active case of Covid on the whole reservation. I don't know why these particular young people died, but some leading causes of death in Dewey County, where Eagle Butte is located, are heart disease, diabetes, liver disease, suicide, and accidents. Young people, parents with small children, die at a devastating rate, a spreading grief that touches everyone on the reservation.

And here was LeBeau, a nurse who knew one hundred years of resistance—and who knew what *could* be, with justice and healing—telling it to anyone who would listen. In fact, insisting upon it. We circled back to her house and got out of the car. "That was the tour! Eagle Butte, USA," she said.

About five months later, Marcella LeBeau died of cancer at age 102. She was a nurse until the day she died. She embodied the nursing practice of seeing a person holistically. Her nursing transcended employment. She was nursing when she testified before Congress, asking that the U.S. government revoke the Medals of Honor it awarded to U.S. soldiers who committed the Massacre at Wounded Knee. She was nursing when she asked the schools to support two-spirited people, and she was nursing when she retrieved stolen Lakota artifacts. She was even nursing when she helped me understand these things. She knew that the past and the present are not separate but living in all our bodies.

I thought of LeBeau and her importance to her community as both an elder and as a healer when I spoke to Michelle Drew, CNM, DNP, about her great-grandmother and her grandmother and their places in their community, and what all that meant for the potential of nursing. "I live in the community where I serve," she told me. "So, I walk down the street, and I hear my name being called. And I think that's how midwives were. And I think nursing has that potential."

Drew went on, speaking about the relationship-based essence of midwifery: "And when I think of what I would've wanted, both when I was giving birth and as a mother, it wouldn't necessarily have been a nurse practitioner who could come in and speak to me on the scientific level of all the whys and hows, but someone who wanted to sit down with me and know who I was. 'Yes, please, talk to me all day about which vaccines and what schedule we should do and why. But please also value me as a person. Value us as a family.' Because that's too much of what medicine has *never* done."

That's too much of what medicine has never done. But nurses can be present for the worst things and the best things, moments that defy description or containment. Nurses can know who you are, where you come from, and what you need.

Mark Lazenby, PhD, APRN, puts it this way: "Nursing is a profoundly radical profession that calls society to equality and justice, to trustworthiness and to openness. The profession is, also, radically political: it imagines a world in which the conditions necessary for health are enjoyed by all people."

Whether you are a nurse or not, imagine it. Imagine a world in which the conditions necessary for health are enjoyed by all people. Nurses have a unique ability to bring such a world to fruition, if they choose it. The rest of us can help: We are not nurses, but we can remember that Neolithic boy whose vertebrae fused as he grew, whose community, nevertheless, didn't let him die of starvation or infection. We can do that, too. We can refuse to be ruled by the dark logic of domination, some cruel fantasy of survival of the fittest. We can choose something different: we can look to ethical nursing, and we can emulate it.

I carry in my body the transformative nursing care I have received. We can carry it; we can multiply it; we can pass it on.

ACKNOWLEDGMENTS

A book is a group project, and I'm so grateful to everyone who made this one possible. First, thank you to my brilliant and steadfast editor, Gail Winston, who never fails to remind me that the reader should be at the center of everything we do in publishing. It has been my privilege to work with such a sharp and thoughtful editor. Thank you to my agent, Jonah Straus, who is generous in so many ways: with his time, knowledge, and enthusiasm. Thank you to editor Sarah Haugen, who jumped in with utter grace and acumen to bring the book to the finish line. Thank you, Gail, Jonah, and Sarah, for believing in these ideas.

So many people—nurses, historians, patients, and family members—took the time to speak with me, to share their knowledge and insight. You'll find many of these people in this book, but not all. Either way, the book benefited from what they shared with me. I'm humbled by your trust. For letting me carry some of your stories and insight, thank you to: the late Marcella LeBeau and to Gerri LeBeau, Cassandra Alexander, Paula N. Kagan, Marie Manthey, Monica McLemore, Teddie M. Potter, Patrick McMurray, Julie Jenkins, Nancy Leftenant-Colon, Cleo Silvers, Monica H. Green, Charissa J. Threat, Kylie M. Smith, Patricia D'Antonio, Stephen and Karen Wickham, Lee Kent, Ginger Brooks, Tobi Ash, Tim Boon, Sarah Creed, Jerry

Soucy, Mariana Sandarovscaia, Nealy Zimmermann, Michelle Drew, Shawna Butler, Liz Stokes, Jonathan Bartels, Melody Butler, Laurie G. Combe, Charlene Kizior, Ashley Bartholomew, Amie Archibald-Varley, Sara Fung, Nezahualcoyotl Xiuhtecutli, India Walton, Tarik S. Khan, Mary Nasuta, Roxana Chicas, Katie Huffling, Jessica LeClair, Christy Haas-Howard, Darcy Jones, Anna Brown, L. Synn Stern, Jason Fox, Phara Souffrant Forrest, Gerard Brogan, Jen Lovallo, Pia Marie Winters Jordan, Michelle Mahon, Zenei Triunfo-Cortez, Shannan, Erin, Stephanie, Cortney, and Tiffany, and "Hannah," and the late "Ahmad."

Thanks also to Estefany and Michelle of the Lantana Collective, who interpreted Spanish for me so I could speak with study participants; and to Melissa Shriver at the Milwaukee Public Library and research librarians at the New York Public Library, who turned up gold. Gratitude and appreciation to Roseline Jean Louis who gave the manuscript a nurse's read.

None of us do this alone: I'm lucky to have brilliant and generous writers and readers as my closest friends. Thank you for diving in with me, Maria Luisa Tucker, Suzanne Cope, Yaran Noti, and Michelle Rome. Thank you so much to the team at Harper: Hayley Salmon, Kate D'Esmond, Katie O'Callaghan, designer Robin Bilardello, and everyone else in the production, design, marketing, editorial, and publicity departments, essential professionals all.

Thank you for your love and support, Jyotsna and Anil Mhatre, Jenny Hellman, Colette Eastwood, Erin Eastwood, and Sharlene Cochrane. And to my family, Amol and Mira (and Buzz and Lola), thanks for listening. I love you.

NOTES

AUTHOR'S NOTE

x   defined, licensed, or delineated: Leigh Whaley, *Women and the Practice of Medical Care in Early Modern Europe, 1400–1800* (New York: Palgrave Macmillan, 2016), 112–13. "The reality is that nurses have always provided the majority of the hands-on care given to sick people, and that the nursing and medical professions share a long history of similar functions and tasks."

INTRODUCTION

xvii she was working within several facets of nursing: American Nurses Association, "What Is Nursing?" ANA, www.nursingworld.org/practice-policy/workforce/what-is-nursing/.

xvii And by calming me: Peter Callery, "Caring for Parents of Hospitalized Children: A Hidden Area of Nursing Work," *Journal of Advanced Nursing* 26, no. 5 (1997): 992–98, PMID: 9372405.

xvii hospitalized kids may have better outcomes: Stephanie K. Doupnik et al., "Parent Coping Support Interventions During Acute Pediatric Hospitalizations: A Meta-Analysis," *Pediatrics* 140, no. 3 (2017): doi.org/10.1542/peds.2016-4171.

    Bernadette Mazurek Melnyk, "Intervention Studies Involving Parents of Hospitalized Young Children: An Analysis of the Past and Future Recommendations," *Journal of Pediatric Nursing* 15, no. 1 (2000): 4–13, https://pubmed.ncbi.nlm.nih.gov/10714033/.

xviii made them feel: This is often attributed to Maya Angelou but the actual provenance of the quote is uncertain.

xix An old vaudeville catcall is "Hello, Nurse!": "Hello Nurse (Vaudeville)," Academic Dictionaries and Encyclopedias, en-academic.com/dic.nsf /enwiki/2432430/.

xix Many of the competing nurse stereotypes are misogynistic: Annette M. Jinks and Eleanor Bradley, "Angel, Handmaiden, Battleaxe or Whore? A Study Which Examines Changes in Newly Recruited Student Nurses' Attitudes to Gender and Nursing Stereotypes," *Nurse Education Today* 24, no. 2 (2004): 121–27, doi.org/10.1016/j.nedt.2003.10.011.

xix most populous profession in the world: Mark Lazenby, *Toward a Better World: The Social Significance of Nursing* (New York: Oxford University Press, 2020), 7.

xix more than 27 million professional nurses and midwives: World Health Organization, *State of the World's Nursing 2020: Investing in Education, Jobs, and Leadership* (Geneva: World Health Organization, 2020), www .who.int/publications/i/item/9789240003279.

xix nurses constitute the largest group: World Health Organization, *State of the World's Nursing 2020*; and American Association of Colleges of Nursing, "Nursing Fact Sheet," AACN, April 1, 2019, www.aacnnursing .org/News-Information/Fact-Sheets/Nursing-Fact-Sheet.

xix three times as many registered nurses: American Association of Colleges of Nursing, "Nursing Fact Sheet."

xx About sixty thousand nurses have doctorates: American Association of Colleges of Nursing, "Number of People Receiving Nursing Doctoral Degrees Annually," Campaign for Action, September 15, 2021, campaignforaction.org/resource/number-people-receiving-nursing -doctoral-degrees-annually/.

xx about five hundred thousand: Adding the numbers from the American Association of Nurse Practitioners (AANP), the National Board of Certification and Recertification for Nurse Anesthetists (NBCRNA), the National Association of Clinical Nurse Specialists (NACNS), and the American College of Nurse-Midwives (ACNM). American Association of Nurse Practitioners, "NP Fact Sheet," American Association of Nurse Practitioners, April 2022, www.aanp.org/about/all-about-nps/np-fact -sheet; American College of Nurse-Midwives, "Fact Sheet: Essential Facts About Midwives," ACNM, June 2021, www.midwife.org/acnm/files/cc libraryfiles/filename/000000008273/EssentialFactsAboutMidwives _Final_June_2021_new.pdf; the National Board of Certification and

Recertification for Nurse Anesthetists, "History: About the NBCRNA," NBCRNA, n.d., www.nbcrna.com/about-us/history; National Association of Clinical Nurse Specialists, "Clinical Nurse Specialists Inspire, Innovate, and Influence," NACNS, May 4, 2018, nacns.org/2018/05/clinical-nurse-specialists-inspire-innovate-and-influence/.

xx   APRNs include: National Council of State Boards of Nursing. "APRNs in the U.S." NCSBN, n.d., www.ncsbn.org/aprn.htm.

xx   they must work under physician "supervision": American Association of Nurse Practitioners, "State Practice Environment," AANP, April 15, 2022, www.aanp.org/advocacy/state/state-practice-environment.

xx   more than four million RNs in the United States: National Council of State Boards of Nursing, "Active RN Licenses," NCSBN, www.ncsbn.org/6161.htm.

xx   About 80 percent identify as: All demographic statistics from Richard A. Smiley et al., "The 2020 National Nursing Workforce Survey," *Journal of Nursing Regulation* 12, no. 1 (2021): S5. doi.org/10.1016/S2155-8256(21)00027-2.

xx   they must pass a licensing test: U.S. Bureau of Labor Statistics, "Licensed Practical and Licensed Vocational Nurses," in *Occupational Outlook Handbook*, U.S. Bureau of Labor Statistics, April 18, 2022, www.bls.gov/ooh/healthcare/licensed-practical-and-licensed-vocational-nurses.htm#tab-4.

xx   practical nurses number about 940,000: Smiley et al., "The 2020 National Nursing Workforce Survey."

xx   more likely than RNs to be people of color: Smiley et al., "The 2020 National Nursing Workforce Survey."

xx   number about 1.4 million: U.S. Bureau of Labor Statistics, "Nursing Assistants and Orderlies," in *Occupational Outlook Handbook*, U.S. Bureau of Labor Statistics, April 18, 2022, www.bls.gov/ooh/healthcare/nursing-assistants.htm.

xx   women of color make up the majority: Manisha Sengupta, Farida K. Ejaz, and Lauren D. Harris-Kojetin, "Training of Home Health Aides and Nurse Aides: Findings from National Data," *Gerontology and Geriatrics Education* 33, no. 4 (2012): 391, doi.org/10.1080/02701960.2012.702167.

xx   median annual salary for a CNA is $30,000: U.S. Bureau of Labor Statistics, "Nursing Assistants and Orderlies."

xx   median annual salary for an RN is $77,000: U.S. Bureau of Labor Statistics, "Registered Nurses," in *Occupational Outlook Handbook*.

xxi   in theory at least: Paula N. Kagan, PhD, RN; Peggy L. Chinn, PhD, RN, FAAN, "We're All Here for the Good of the Patient: A Dialogue on Power," December 21, 2009, doi.org/10.1177/0894318409353808.

xxi   duty to assess and care for each patient holistically: "NCLEX-RN Exam Guide," Registered Nursing, April 15, 2022, www.registerednursing.org/nclex/#category-3-psychosocial-integrity.

xxi   within a family, a community, or an environment: American Nurses Association, "What Is Nursing?"

xxii   If you are being discharged: Janice B. Foust, "Discharge Planning as Part of Daily Nursing Practice," *Applied Nursing Research* 20, no. 2 (2007): 72–77, doi.org/10.1016/j.apnr.2006.01.005.

xxiii   difference between medicine and nursing: Cassandra Alexander, *Year of the Nurse: A Covid-19 2020 Pandemic Memoir* (Caskara Press, 2021), 21.

xxiii   Another part of a nurse's job is to advocate: Lois Gerber, "Understanding the Nurse's Role as a Patient Advocate," *Nursing* 48, no. 4 (2018): 55–58, doi.org/10.1097/01.nurse.0000531007.02224.65.

xxiv   Paula N. Kagan, PhD, RN: Paula Kagan, phone interview with author, April 17, 2020.

xxv   therapeutic value in the connection between nurse and patient: Marie Manthey et al., "Primary Nursing: A Return to the Concept of 'My Nurse' and 'My Patient,'" *Nursing Forum* 9, no. 1 (1970): 65–84, doi.org/10.1111/j.1744-6198.1970.tb00442.x.

xxv   model of primary care was co-developed: Riane Eisler et al., *Transforming Interprofessional Partnerships: A New Framework for Nursing and Partnership-Based Health Care* (Indianapolis, IN: Sigma Theta Tau International, 2014), 216.

xxv   "I felt abandoned": Marie Manthey, author phone interview, September 28, 2020.

xxv   Monica McLemore, PhD, RN: Monica McLemore, author phone interview, September 16, 2020.

xxvi   "good moral character": Office of the Professions, "License Requirements: Registered Professional Nursing," NYSED, June 22, 2022, www.op.nysed.gov/prof/nurse/nursingrn.htm.

xxvi   ancient India: Agniveśa Caraka et al., *Caraka-Saṃhitā: Agniveśa's*

Treatise Refined and Annotated by Caraka and Redacted by Dṛḍha-bala: Text with English Translation (Varanasi: Chaukhambha Orientalia, 2014.)

xxvi   "The moral character of nursing": Mark Lazenby, *Caring Matters Most: The Ethical Significance of Nursing* (New York: Oxford University Press, 2017), 5–6.

xxvii   30 seconds before they interrupt them: Naykky Singh Ospina et al., "Eliciting the Patient's Agenda: Secondary Analysis of Recorded Clinical Encounters," *Journal of General Internal Medicine* 34, no. 1 (2018): 36, https://doi.org/10.1007/s11606-018-4540-5.

xxviii   As Potter explained: Teddie M. Potter, PhD, author Zoom interview, August 3, 2021.

xxviii   a staggering 92 percent of Black nurses: All statistics in this paragraph are from American Nurses Association, "New Survey Data: Racism Within the Nursing Profession Is a Substantial Problem," ANA, January 25, 2022, www.nursingworld.org/news/news-releases/2021/new -survey-data-racism-in-nursing/.

xxviii   make registered nursing less disproportionately white: Julia Cusick et al., "How to Ease the Nursing Shortage in America," Center for American Progress, June 7, 2022, www.americanprogress.org/article/how-to -ease-the-nursing-shortage-in-america/.

xxviii   more likely to come from Black or brown or low-income: E. Mahaffey, "The Relevance of Associate Degree Nursing Education: Past, Present, Future," Online Journal of Issues in Nursing 7, no. 2 (2002): https:// ojin.nursingworld.org/MainMenuCategories/ANAMarketplace/ANA Periodicals/OJIN/TableofContents/Volume72002/No2May2002 /RelevanceofAssociateDegree.html.

xxix   many hospitals are phasing out: "The Future of the Associate Degree in Nursing Program," NursingLicensure, February 2, 2022, www.nurs inglicensure.org/articles/adn-program-future/.

xxix   more likely to work in underserved areas: Erin Fraher, PhD, MPP, "The Nursing Workforce: Trends and Challenges," The Cecil G. Sheps Center for Health Services Research, www.shepscenter.unc.edu/wp -content/uploads/2016/09/Fraher_NCGenAssembly_Mar2016.pdf.

xxix   Patrick McMurray, MSN, RN: Patrick McMurray, author phone interview, July 7, 2020.

xxix   disproportionate bars: "New RN Graduates by Degree Type, by Race

/Ethnicity," Campaign for Action, June 17, 2022, campaignforaction .org/resource/new-rn-graduates-degree-type-raceethnicity/.

xxix operates from a harmful sense of scarcity: Nadia Primc, "Dealing with Scarcity of Resources in Nursing: The Scope and Limits of Individual Responsibility," *European Journal for Nursing History and Ethics* 2 (2020), www.enhe.eu/archive/2020/5054.

xxix nurse staffing shortages: American Association of Colleges of Nursing, "NursingShortage,"AACN,September2020,www.aacnnursing.org/news -information/fact-sheets/nursing-shortage.

xxix brought about by poor working conditions: Lucy King and Jonah Kessel, "We Know the Real Cause of the Crisis in Our Hospitals. It's Greed." *New York Times*, January 19, 2022, www.nytimes.com/video/opinion /100000008158650/covid-nurse-burnout-understaffing.html.

xxix A new national survey: National Nurses United, "National Nurse Survey Reveals Significant Increases in Unsafe Staffing, Workplace Violence, and Moral Distress," NNU, April 14, 2022, www.nationalnursesunited .org/press/survey-reveals-increases-in-unsafe-staffing-workplace -violence-moral-distress.

xxix Sixty-two percent of nurses: Christine T. Kovner et al., "Newly Licensed RNs' Characteristics, Work Attitudes, and Intentions to Work," *American Journal of Nursing* 107, no. 9 (2007): 58, doi.org/10.1097/01.naj .0000287512.31006.66.

xxx "As some nursing moved out of the realm": Susan M. Reverby, *Ordered to Care: The Dilemma of American Nursing, 1850–1945* (Cambridge, UK: Cambridge University Press, 2004), 2.

xxx Julie Jenkins, DNP, APRN: Julie Jenkins, author phone interview, March 16, 2022.

CHAPTER 1: ORIGINS

2 These are interactions: Margaret Mead supposedly cited evidence of a healed broken femur as the first sign of "civilization," but this is unverified and likely untrue. See Gideon Lasco, "Did Margaret Mead Think a Healed Femur Was the Earliest Sign of Civilization?" SAPIENS, June 15, 2022, www.sapiens.org/column/entanglements/margaret-mead-femur/.

2 Klippel-Feil syndrome: U.S. Department of Health and Human Services, "Klippel-Feil Syndrome," National Institute of Neurological Disorders and Stroke, April 25, 2022, www.ninds.nih.gov/health-information

/disorders/klippel-feil-syndrome#:~:text=Publications-,Definition, early%20weeks%20of%20fetal%20development.

2   would have died within days: Information over the next several paragraphs about this case and Lorna Tilley's work is from the following sources: Marc F. Oxenham et al., "Paralysis and Severe Disability Requiring Intensive Care in Neolithic Asia," *Anthropological Science* 117, no. 2 (2009): 107–12, doi.org/10.1537/ase.081114; Lorna Tilley, "The Bioarcheology of Care," *The SAA Archaeological Record* 12, no. 3 (May 2012): 39–41; Andrew Curry, "Ancient Bones Offer Clues to How Long Ago Humans Cared for the Vulnerable," National Public Radio, WAMU, June 17, 2020, wamu.org/story/20/06/17/ancient-bones-offer-clues-to -how-long-ago-humans-cared-for-the-vulnerable/.

3   spina bifida: Boyce Rensberger, "Florida Bog Reveals 8,000-Year-Old Secrets," *Washington Post*, October 26, 1986, https://www.washington post.com/archive/politics/1986/10/26/florida-bog-reveals-8000-year -old-secrets/efaacbdf-0b89–42a8–841a-8cf16e8dd72e/.

3   The skeleton of a young woman: Alecia Schrenk and Lorna Tilley, "Caring in Ancient Times," *Anthropology News* 59, no. 1 (January 2018), e59-e60: doi.org/10.1111/an.743.

3   previous archeological studies: Tilley, "The Bioarcheology of Care," 39–41.

3   "Our past contains important lessons for our present": Schrenk and Tilley, "Caring in Ancient Times," e62.

4   tales of domination, empire building, and violence: For more on how domination and partnership paradigms affect nursing power and practice, see Eisler et al., *Transforming Interprofessional Partnerships*.

4   nursing historians have painstakingly excavated: Historians whose work has been instrumental in the research of this book include Charissa J. Threat, PhD; Patricia D'Antonio, PhD RN; Sara Ritchey, PhD; Kylie M. Smith, PhD; Jean C. Whelan, PhD, RN; Deborah Gray White, PhD; Carol Helmstadter, RN; Sharon T. Strocchia, PhD; Monica H. Green, PhD; Darlene Clark Hine, PhD; Stephanie Y. Mitchem, PhD; Sharla M. Fett, PhD; Leigh Whaley, PhD; and Guenter B. Risse, PhD.

4   "In attempting to study the history of nursing": Adelaide M. Nutting and Lavinia L. Dock, *A History of Nursing: The Evolution of Nursing Systems from Earliest Times to the Foundation of the First English and American Training Schools for Nurses* (New York: Putnam, 1907), 7.

5   "Nursing has a long and rich history": Sameh Elhabashy and Elsha-
     imaa M. Abdelgawad, "The History of Nursing Profession in Ancient
     Egyptian Society," *International Journal of Africa Nursing Sciences* 11
     (2019): 100174, doi.org/10.1016/j.ijans.2019.100174.

5   the sole founder of modern nursing: "Florence Nightingale," History
     .com, November 9, 2009, www.history.com/topics/womens-history/flor
     ence-nightingale-1; Wikipedia, n.d., en.wikipedia.org/wiki/Florence
     _Nightingale.

5   like most lone-hero narratives, this one is not entirely true: I was also
     under this impression when I began researching this book. Emory Uni-
     versity historian Kylie M. Smith, PhD, was one of the first to point out
     to me that it was impossible for one person to have invented modern
     nursing.

5   venerable group of German deaconess nurses: Natasha McEnroe, "Cele-
     brating Florence Nightingale's Bicentenary," *The Lancet* 395, no. 10235
     (2020): 1475–78, https://doi.org/10.1016/S0140-6736(20)30992-2.

6   a profession for well-off white women: Natalie Stake-Doucet, "The Rac-
     ist Lady with the Lamp," *Nursing Clio* (blog), November 29, 2021,
     nursingclio.org/2020/11/05/the-racist-lady-with-the-lamp/.

6   "practiced by mothers and handed down": Leigh Whaley, "Motherly
     Medicine," in her *Women and the Practice of Medical Care in Early
     Modern Europe, 1400–1800* (Houndmills, Basingstoke, UK: Palgrave
     Macmillan, 2011), chap. 8, 150.

6   Follow these threads back more than two thousand years: "Charaka-
     Samhita," Britannica, www.britannica.com/topic/Charaka-samhita.

6   one of ayurveda's major texts: "Origin of Ayurveda," National Health
     Portal, Government of India, May 6, 2015, www.nhp.gov.in/origin-of
     -ayurveda_mtl.

6   without any one of them, health care would not exist: Govind S. Raj-
     poot, *Interpretation of the Charaka Samhita* (Prague: University of
     Ayurveda, 2016), 291–93.

7   "of good behavior, distinguished for purity": Nutting and Dock, *A His-
     tory of Nursing*, 34.

7   a fact often credited to Buddhist emperor Ashoka: F. P. Retief and
     L. Cilliers, "The Evolution of Hospitals from Antiquity to the Renais-
     sance," *Acta Theologica* 26, no. 2 (2010), 216: doi.org/10.4314/actat.v2
     6i2.52575.

7   the pursuit of righteousness: Amulya Chandra Sen, "Ashoka," Britannica, www.britannica.com/biography/Ashoka; Kristin Baird Rattini, "Who Was Ashoka?" National Geographic, May 4, 2021, www.nationalgeographic.com/culture/article/ashoka?loggedin=true.

7   both physicians and nurses tended to patients: Rajpoot, *Interpretation of the Charaka Samhita*, 291–93.

7   around 250 BCE: Chad E. O'Lynn and Russell E. Tranbarger, "History of Men in Nursing: A Review," in their *Men in Nursing: History, Challenges, and Opportunities* (New York: Springer, 2007), 9; Tamsin Smith, "'Nursing History Goes Beyond Nightingale,'" RCN Magazines, June 1, 2021, www.rcn.org.uk/magazines/opinion/2021/june/nursing-history-goes-beyond-nightingale.

8   trained nursing that made it possible: Information in this paragraph is from Nutting and Dock, *A History of Nursing*, 34; and Retief and Cilliers, "The Evolution of Hospitals from Antiquity to the Renaissance," 216.

8   a sign of her importance and the intimacy of their relationship: For the information in this paragraph, see Elhabashy and Abdelgawad, "The History of Nursing Profession in Ancient Egyptian Society,"; and Carolyn Graves-Brown, "Women's Work," in her *Dancing for Hathor: Women in Ancient Egypt* (New York: Bloomsbury, 2013), chap. 5, 83.

8   hard to win wars and maintain control without nurses: Guenter B. Risse, "Pre-Christian Healing Places: Collective Care of Soldiers and Slaves: Roman Valetudinaria," in his *Mending Bodies, Saving Souls: A History of Hospitals* (New York: Oxford University Press, 1999), chap. 1, 38–59.

9   called *valetudinaria*: Risse, "Pre-Christian Healing Places," 38–59.

9   up to five hundred patients: Valentine Belfiglio, "Perioperative Anesthesia in Ancient Rome: 27 BC–AD 476," *Neurology and Neuroscience Reports* 1, no. 1 (2018): doi.org/10.15761/nnr.1000101.

9   from 115 CE: Risse, "Pre-Christian Healing Places," 38.

9   box containing bandages: Risse, "Pre-Christian Healing Places," 50.

9   ancient Greek theory of the four humors: Risse, "Pre-Christian Healing Places," 53.

9   accepted throughout the West for more than two thousand years: Faith Lagay, "The Legacy of Humoral Medicine," *Journal of Ethics American Medical Association*, July 1, 2002, https://journalofethics.ama-assn.org/article/legacy-humoral-medicine/2002-07.

9   *capsarii* used vinegar to wash wounds: Surajit Bhattacharya, "Wound Healing Through the Ages," *Indian Journal of Plastic Surgery* 45, no. 2 (2012): 177-79, http://doi.org/10.4103/0970-0358.101255.

9   honey to prevent infection: Belfiglio, "Perioperative Anesthesia in Ancient Rome: 27 BC-AD 476."

10 administered opium for pain: Belfiglio, "Perioperative Anesthesia in Ancient Rome: 27 BC-AD 476."

10 Rufaida Al-Aslamiya grew up: Rafat Jan, "Rufaida Al-Aslamiya, the First Muslim Nurse," *Image: The Journal of Nursing Scholarship* 28, no. 3 (1996): 267-68, https://doi.org/10.1111/j.1547-5069.1996.tb00362.x.

10 Muhammad embarked on a series of battles: Jan, "Rufaida Al-Aslamiya, the First Muslim Nurse," 267.

10 provided drinking water and food: For information on her wartime nursing practice, see Jan, "Rufaida Al-Aslamiya, the First Muslim Nurse," 267-68; and Samar Yahya, "Rufaida Al-Aslamia—the First Muslim Nurse," *Saudi Gazette*, March 31, 2017, saudigazette.com.sa/article /175811.

10 Rufaida was able to remove an arrow: Omar Hasan Kasule Sr., "Historical Roots of the Nursing Profession in Islam," Paper Presented at the Third International Nursing Conference, Empowerment and Health: An Agenda for Nurses in the Twenty-first Century, held in Brunei, Dar as Salam, November 1-4, 1998, web.archive.org/web/20020214083140 /http://www.iiu.edu.my/medic/islmed/Lecmed/rufaid98.nov.html.

11 championing preventative care and education: Jan, "Rufaida Al-Aslamiya, the First Muslim Nurse," 267.

11 who has studied Rufaida: Kasule, "Historical Roots of the Nursing Profession in Islam."

11 a precursor to nursing discharge planning: For the information in this paragraph, see "Islamic Culture and the Medical Arts: Hospitals," U.S. National Library of Medicine, National Institutes of Health, December 15, 2011, www.nlm.nih.gov/exhibition/islamic_medical/islamic_12 .html.

12 who tried to save her father's life: Leigh Whaley, "The Medieval Contribution," in her *Women and the Practice of Medical Care in Early Modern Europe, 1400-1800* (UK edition), chap. 1, 8-10.

12 a worried Anna took charge of his care: For details on the last days of Alexius and on Anna's care, see Anna Komnene, "Last Illness and Death

of Alexius," Book XV of *The Alexiad*, Internet History Sourcebooks, sourcebooks.fordham.edu/basis/AnnaComnena-Alexiad15.asp.

13   the oldest kind of nurse: Whaley, "The Medieval Contribution," 8-10.

13   only a fraction of medieval female practitioners: Monica Green, "Women's Medical Practice and Health Care in Medieval Europe," *Signs: Journal of Women in Culture and Society* 14, no. 2 (1989):444-45, doi .org/10.1086/494516.

13   particularly male physicians: Kamber L. Hart, AB, "Trends in Proportion of Women as Authors of Medical Journal Articles, 2008-2018," *JAMA Internal Medicine* 179, no. 9 (September 2019): 1285-87, jamanet work.com/journals/jamainternalmedicine/fullarticle/2733558#:~:text =In%20the%20274%20764%20articles,7.8%25%20from%202008%20 to%202018.

13   built the Pantokrator: Vern L. Bullough and Bonnie Bullough, "Medieval Nursing," *Nursing History Review* 1, no. 1 (1993): 89-104, https:// doi.org/10.1891/1062-8061.1.1.89.

13   one of the most advanced hospitals of the time: Though early modern European hospitals are often cited as the precursors to the modern hospital, some scholars argue that Byzantine hospitals are the closer comparisons. For instance, see Timothy S. Miller, *Birth of the Hospital in the Byzantine Empire* (Baltimore, MD: Johns Hopkins University Press, 1997).

14   nursing staff of about forty-six was permanent: Guenter B. Risse, "Church and Laity: Partnership in Hospital Care: The Pantocrator Xenon of Constantinople," in his *Mending Bodies, Saving Souls: A History of Hospitals*, chap. 3, 126.

14   made up of professionals: Lambrini Kourkouta, "Working Conditions and Duties of Nurses in Byzantium," *International History of Nursing Journal* 4, no. 1 (February 1998): 32-34.

14   the two sexes earned the same wage: For details on the Pantokrator and the roles of nurses and physicians, see Bullough and Bullough, "Medieval Nursing," 93-5; and Pan Codellas, "The Pantocrator, the Imperial Byzantine Medical Center of Century AD in Constantinople," JSTOR, *Bulletin of the History of Medicine* 12, no. 2 (July 1942): 392-410, www .jstor.org/stable/44446279.

14   "God hit me with a painful sore through the whole body": For information on Prodromos's illness and hospitalization, see Risse, "Church and

Laity: Partnership in Hospital Care: The Pantocrator Xenon of Constan-tinople," 130–34.

15   Phoebe, a deaconess in the New Testament: "The Origins and Meaning of Nursing," Sacred Heart University, July 25, 2020, onlineprograms .sacredheart.edu/resources/article/the-origins-and-meaning-of-nursing/.

15   Monasteries and convents lent themselves: Leigh Whaley, "The Healing Care of Nurses," in her *Women and the Practice of Medical Care in Early Modern Europe, 1400–1800* (New York edition), chap. 6, 113–17.

16   visited people at home to care for them: This paragraph is from Whaley, "The Healing Care of Nurses," 115–19.

16   Black Death plague of the 1300s: Michael S. Rosenwald, "History's Dead-liest Pandemics, from Ancient Rome to Modern America," *Washington Post*, October 3, 2021, www.washingtonpost.com/graphics/2020/local /retropolis/coronavirus-deadliest-pandemics/.

16   Many nuns and monks died while nursing others: Jennifer Viegas, "Re-naissance Nuns Wiped Out by Plague," NBC News, February 6, 2009, www.nbcnews.com/id/wbna29054365.

16   workers excavated a mass grave on the site: Hugh Willmott et al., "A Black Death Mass Grave at Thornton Abbey: The Discovery and Ex-amination of a Fourteenth-Century Rural Catastrophe," *Antiquity* 94, no. 373 (2020): 179–96, doi.org/10.15184/aqy.2019.213.

16   work of religious women in the late Middle Ages: Sara Ritchey, *Acts of Care: Recovering Women in Late Medieval Health* (Ithaca, NY: Cornell University Press, 2021), 2.

17   health matters of all kinds: Sharon T. Strocchia, "The Business of Health: Convent Pharmacies in Renaissance Italy," in her *Forgotten Healers: Women and the Pursuit of Health in Late Renaissance Italy* (Cambridge, MA: Harvard University Press, 2019), chap. 3, 130–78.

17   *Forgotten Healers*: Historian Kylie M. Smith, PhD, first pointed me to this book.

17   Among the jars and vials: All details in this paragraph are from Stroc-chia, *Forgotten Healers*, 101–09.

18   Beguines: "Beguines," Britannica, www.britannica.com/topic/Beguines.

18   "Her therapeutic actions were recorded": Ritchey, *Acts of Care*, 1–2.

18   practical and hands-on: Bullough and Bullough, "Medieval Nursing," 98–99.

18   nun apothecaries often included reassuring "proofs": Sharon Strocchia, "Gifts of Health," in her *Forgotten Healers*, chap. 4, 164.

19   "In this view, human life is understood": This paragraph is from Stephanie Y. Mitchem, *African American Folk Healing* (New York: New York University Press, 2007), 33.

19   Enslaved people practiced nursing care: Sharla M. Fett, "Doctoring Women," in her *Working Cures: Healing, Health, and Power on Southern Slave Plantations (Gender and American Culture)* (Chapel Hill: University of North Carolina Press, 2002), chap. 5, 111–41; Deborah Gray White, "The Female Slave Network," in *Ar'n't I a Woman?: Female Slaves in the Plantation South* (New York: W. W. Norton, 1999), 119–41.

19   in both Black and white communities: Darlene Clark Hine, "Origins of the Black Hospital and Nurse Training School Movement: An Overview," in her *Black Women in White: Racial Conflict and Cooperation in the Nursing Profession, 1890–1950 (Blacks in the Diaspora)* (Bloomington: Indiana University Press, 1989), chap. 1, 3.

19   accused of poisoning the child if they died: Fett, *Working Cures*, chap. 6, 160.

20   washed the dead: Sharla M. Fett, "Sacred Plants," in her *Working Cures*, chap. 3, 60–83.

20   cautions against romanticizing this kind of work: Dorothy E. Roberts, "Reproduction Is Bondage," in her *Killing the Black Body: Race, Reproduction, and the Meaning of Liberty* (New York: Vintage, 1999), chap. 1, 54.

20   Minor was set free in 1825: The Jensey Snow/Jane Minor information is from Hine, "Origins of the Black Hospital and Nurse Training School Movement: An Overview," 3; and Stacy H. Adams, "Jane Minor," *Richmond Times-Dispatch*, February 23, 1999, richmond.com /jane-minor/article_5328088c-6b14-11e2-811f-001a4bcf6878.html.

CHAPTER 2: HIERARCHY

23   that says physicians are the only heroes: Bullough and Bullough, "Medieval Nursing," 101.

24   skills could be gained through family or apprenticeship: Historian Monica H. Green, PhD, explained: "The early 12th century was the

last moment in Western history when there were no legal restrictions whatsoever on medical practice. Just as in Antiquity, the 'medical marketplace' was open to anyone who wished to lay claim to medical expertise." Green, *Making Women's Medicine Masculine: The Rise of Male Authority in Pre-Modern Gynaecology* (Oxford: Oxford University Press, 2009), 3.

24 University of Salerno: de Divitiis, Enrico, Paolo Cappabianca, and Oreste de Divitiis, "The 'Schola Medica Salernitana': The Forerunner of the Modern University Medical Schools," *Neurosurgery* 55, no. 4 (2004): 722–45. doi.org/10.1227/01.neu.0000139458.36781.31.

24 in a legal gray area: Bullough and Bullough, "Medieval Nursing" 100; Whaley, "The Healing Care of Nurses," 113.

25 "exclusion of women from the universities": Bullough and Bullough, "Medieval Nursing," 99.

25 women were forbidden from providing medical care: Green, "Women's Medical Practice and Health Care in Medieval Europe," 447.

26 not very many of them at first: Bullough and Bullough, "Medieval Nursing," 98.

26 centuries-long campaign to invent: Green, "Women's Medical Practice and Health Care in Medieval Europe," 458. Green writes of the physician's attempts "to construct a social distinction between himself and a 'lower' class of healers who in reality practice a medicine not so very different from his own."

26 "One way that physicians sought to distinguish": Sara Ritchey, "Women Were the Unseen Healthcare Providers of the Middle Ages," *Aeon*, October 12, 2021, aeon.co/essays/women-were-the-unseen-healthcare -providers-of-the-middle-ages.

26 Jacoba Felicie: I first discovered the story of this trial through the writings of Monica H. Green.

26 brought Felicie to court and accused her: All details from the court case are from the translation in Chartulary of the University of Paris, "The Case of a Woman Doctor in Paris," in James Bruce Ross and Mary Martin McLaughlin, eds., *The Portable Medieval Reader* (New York: Viking Press, 1949), 635–40.

27 She was fined sixty livres and excommunicated: Monica H. Green, "Getting to the Source: The Case of Jacoba Felicie and the Impact of 'The

Portable Medieval Reader' on the Canon of Medieval Women's History," *Medieval Feminist Forum* 42 (2006): 49–62, https://www.researchgate .net/publication/30011458_Getting_to_the_Source_The_Case_of _Jacoba_Felicie_and_the_Impact_of_the_Portable_Medieval_Reader _on_the_Canon_of_Medieval_Women%27s_History.

28 worse than execution: Roselind Hill, "The Theory and Practice of Excommunication in Medieval England," *History* 42, no. 144 (1957): 1–11, https://doi.org/10.1111/j.1468-229x.1957.tb02266.x.

29 until she died, nine years later: All information on Sister Orsola from Strocchia, "Gifts of Health," 67–84.

29 in the 1300s: Livia Gershon, "Where Witch Hunts Began," JSTOR Daily, June 23, 2018, daily.jstor.org/where-witch-hunts-began/.

29 macabre fantasies about midwives: W. L. Minkowski, "Women Healers of the Middle Ages: Selected Aspects of Their History," *American Journal of Public Health* 82, no. 2 (1992): 288–95, doi.org/10.2105 /ajph.82.2.288.

30 The *Malleus Maleficarum*: Heinrich Institoris and Jakob Sprenger, trans. Christopher S. Mackay, *Malleus Maleficarum* (Cambridge, UK: Cambridge University Press, 2011).

30 "Even an innocent midwife": Minkowski, "Women Healers of the Middle Ages," 294.

30 Scotland saw a disproportionately high: *Newes from Scotland*, witchcraft pamphlet, British Library, www.bl.uk/collection-items/witchcraft -pamphlet-news-from-scotland-1591.

30 Scottish midwife Agnes Sampson: Harley, "Historians as Demonologists," 14.

30 strangled to death before being burned: Julian Goodare, "A Royal Obsession with Black Magic Started Europe's Most Brutal Witch Hunts," *National Geographic*, October 17, 2019, www.nationalgeographic.co.uk /history-and-civilisation/2019/10/royal-obsession-black-magic-started -europes-most-brutal-witch.

30 an instance: Goodare, "A Royal Obsession with Black Magic Started Europe's Most Brutal Witch Hunts."

31 Paula de Eguiluz: Diana Lyn Baptiste et al., "Hidden Figures of Nursing: The Historical Contributions of Black Nurses and a Narrative for Those Who Are Unnamed, Undocumented, and Underrepresented,"

Journal of Advanced Nursing 77, no. 4 (2021): 1627–32, doi.org/10.1111/jan.14791.

32 intoned her crimes: All details on de Eguiluz are from Erica Ball, Tatiana Seijas, and Terri L. Snyder, eds., "Paula De Eguiluz, Seventeenth-Century Puerto Rico, Cuba, and New Grenada (Colombia)," in their *As If She Were Free: A Collective Biography of Women and Emancipation in the Americas* (Cambridge, UK: Cambridge University Press, 2020), 43–57.

32 "De Eguiluz represents": Baptiste et al., "Hidden Figures of Nursing," 1627–32.

33 already a popular and familiar stereotype: Charles Dickens, *The Life and Adventures of Martin Chuzzlewit* (Harmondsworth, UK: Penguin Books, 1968).

33 Bullough write: Bullough and Bullough. "Medieval Nursing," 101.

33 midwives were taking most of the business: Ranana Dine, "Scarlet Letters: Getting the History of Abortion and Contraception Right," Center for American Progress, June 27, 2022, www.americanprogress.org/article/scarlet-letters-getting-the-history-of-abortion-and-contraception-right/.

33 a now-deleted: "Docs vs NPS, PAS: How AMA Made Scope Creep Fight Uglier," Medscape, December 18, 2020, www.medscape.com/viewarticle/941987?reg=1vp_1.

34 lobbied against: "AMA Successfully Fights Scope-of-Practice Expansions that Threaten Patient Safety," American Medical Association, n.d., www.ama-assn.org/practice-management/scope-practice/ama-successfully-fights-scope-practice-expansions-threaten.

34 In twenty-four states: American Association of Nurse Practitioners, "State Practice Environment."

34 collaborative practice agreements: Brendan Martin and Maryann Alexander, "The Economic Burden and Practice Restrictions Associated with Collaborative Practice Agreements: A National Survey of Advanced Practice Registered Nurses," *Journal of Nursing Regulation* 9, no. 4 (2019): 22–30, doi.org/10.1016/S2155-8256(19)30012-2.

34 In 2022, Kansas became: Bruce Japsen, "Kansas Lifts Hurdle to Nurse Practitioners, Becomes 26th State to Do So," *Forbes*, April 18, 2022, www.forbes.com/sites/brucejapsen/2022/04/15/kansas-lifts-hurdle-to-nurse-practitioners-becomes-26th-state-to-do-so/?sh=25d33243793f.

34 "reduced safety for patients": Andis Robeznieks, "Why Expanding APRN Scope of Practice Is a Bad Idea," American Medical Association, October 30, 2020, www.ama-assn.org/practice-management/scope-practice /why-expanding-aprn-scope-practice-bad-idea.

35 Randomized clinical trials have shown: Mary O. Mundinger et al., "Primary Care Outcomes in Patients Treated by Nurse Practitioners or Physicians," *JAMA* 283, no. 1 (2000): 59, doi.org/10.1001/jama.283.1.59; and Mona Shattell, "'Mid-Level' and Primary Care 'Providers': Nomenclature that Stings," *HuffPost*, February 18, 2017, www.huffpost.com /entry/mid-level-and-primary-care-providers-nomenclature-that-stings _b_9265618.

35 did not differ in quality, cost, or outcome: Chuan-Fen Liu et al., "Outcomes of Primary Care Delivery by Nurse Practitioners: Utilization, Cost, and Quality of Care," *Health Services Research* 55, no. 2 (2020): 178–89, https://doi.org/10.1111/1475-6773.13246.

35 there *was* a difference: Megan Moldestad, "Comparable, but Distinct: Perceptions of Primary Care Provided by Physicians and Nurse Practitioners in Full and Restricted Practice Authority States," *Journal of Advanced Nursing* 76, no. 11 (2020): 3092–93, doi.org/10.1111/jan.14501.

35 has called for ending physician oversight: Mary K. Wakefield et al., eds., "Scope-of-Practice Restrictions That Reduce the Productive Capacity of Registered Nurses and Nurse Practitioners," in *The Future of Nursing 2020–2030: Charting a Path to Achieve Health Equity* (Washington, DC: The National Academies Press, 2021), 86–89.

36 proposed a reason: Marilyn W. Edmunds, "The AMA Beehive Is Buzzing Again," *The Journal for Nurse Practitioners* 4, no. 8 (2008): 563, doi .org/10.1016/j.nurpra.2008.07.010.

CHAPTER 3: IDENTITY

38 told the *New York Times*: "11 Army Hospitals Arriving in Europe Without Nurses as Volunteers Are Lacking," *New York Times*, February 1, 1945, www.nytimes.com/1945/02/01/archives/11-army-hospitals-arriving -in-europe-without-nurses-as-volunteers.html?searchResultPosition=1.

38 Newly graduated from nursing school: Pia Marie Winters Jordan first told me about Nancy Leftenant-Colon. All quotes from Leftenant-Colon and information about her in this chapter, unless otherwise noted, are from author's in-person interview with Colon, June 22, 2021.

39   the fight to nurse during war: The context and my analysis of race and gender as they pertain to military nursing are both heavily influenced by a telephone interview with historian Charissa J. Threat, PhD, August 12, 2020, and by Threat's book *Nursing Civil Rights: Gender and Race in the Army Nurse Corps* (Urbana: University of Illinois Press, 2015).

40   this weaponized status: Stake-Doucet, "The Racist Lady with the Lamp."

40   said historian: Charissa J. Threat, phone interview with the author, August 12, 2020.

40   "the Black Nightingale": Julia Buss, *Black Nightingale: Mary Seacole, Hero of the Crimean War* (self-pub., 2011).

40   Seacole was born in 1805: Jane Robinson, "A Female Ulysses," in her *The Charismatic Black Nurse Who Became a Heroine of the Crimea* (London: Constable and Robinson, 2006), chap. 1, 1–20.

41   her dolls: Unless otherwise noted, all details and quotes from Seacole in this chapter are from her autobiography, Mary J. Seacole and Sarah Salih, *Wonderful Adventures of Mrs Seacole in Many Lands* (London: Penguin, 2005).

42   the power vacuum: "Crimean War," National Army Museum, n.d., www .nam.ac.uk/explore/crimean-war; and "Crimean War," Britannica, n.d., www.britannica.com/event/Crimean-War.

42   the war would be over soon: In my research for this chapter, I was heavily influenced by Carol Helmstadter's book *Beyond Nightingale*, to which historian Kylie M. Smith, PhD, first pointed me. Carol Helmstadter, *Beyond Nightingale Nursing on the Crimean War Battlefields* (Manchester, UK: Manchester University Press, 2021), 1.

42   so squalid as to be dangerous: Mark Bostridge, "In the Hey-Day of My Power," in his *Florence Nightingale: The Making of an Icon* (New York: Farrar, Straus and Giroux, 2008), chap. 8, 204–5.

44   a woman of her class did not take a paying job: Bostridge, *Florence Nightingale*, 188–91.

44   The *Times* war correspondent in Constantinople wrote: Bostridge, *Florence Nightingale*, 204.

44   the first war with regular photojournalism: Barbara Orbach Natanson, "Witness to History: Roger Fenton's Photographs of the Crimean War," Prints and Photos, Library of Congress, March 23, 2017, blogs.loc.gov

/picturethis/2017/03/witness-to-history-roger-fentons-photographs-of-the-crimean-war/.

45   sterling bearing and upbringing: Details in this and the previous paragraph are from Carol Helmstadter, "British Nursing at the Beginning of the Crimean War," in her *Beyond Nightingale*, chap. 2.

45   Herbert's bigger, more public plan: Bostridge, "In the Hey-Day of My Power," 204–7.

46   be of unimpeachable character: Details in this paragraph are from Helmstadter, *Beyond Nightingale*, chaps. 2 and 3, 31–76.

46   "hell on earth": Dr. Howard Markel, "How Florence Nightingale Cleaned up 'Hell on Earth' Hospitals and Became an International Hero," PBS, May 12, 2017, www.pbs.org/newshour/health/florence-nightingale-cleaned-hell-earth-hospitals-became-international-hero.

47   dirty air and bad odors: Sarah Zhang, "We're Just Rediscovering a 19th-Century Pandemic Strategy," *The Atlantic*, May 4, 2021, www.theatlantic.com/health/archive/2021/02/bad-air/618106/.

47   clean the drains: Elizabeth Fee and Mary E. Garofalo, "Florence Nightingale and the Crimean War," *American Journal of Public Health* 100, no. 9 (2010): 1591, doi.org/10.2105/ajph.2009.188607.

47   about 2 percent: Joshua Hammer, "The Defiance of Florence Nightingale," Smithsonian, March 1, 2020, www.smithsonianmag.com/history/the-worlds-most-famous-nurse-florence-nightingale-180974155/.

47   her original use of statistics: McEnroe, "Celebrating Florence Nightingale's Bicentenary," 1475–78.

47   the importance of ventilation: "Letter from Florence Nightingale Describing the Benefits of Clean Air, 8 September 1860," British Library, n.d., www.bl.uk/collection-items/letter-from-florence-nightingale-describing-the-benefits-of-clean-air.

47   and in a male-dominated war zone: Carol Helmstadter, "Nightingale's Team of Nurses," in her *Beyond Nightingale*, chap. 2, 61–76.

48   into "civilization": Gayle Morris, "Florence Nightingale: Uncovering Her Impacts on Nursing and Colonialism," *Nurse Journal*, February 28, 2022, nursejournal.org/articles/facts-about-florence-nightingale/.

48   "slept with the key under her pillow": All details from this paragraph and the previous one are from Helmstadter, "Nightingale's Team of Nurses," 61–76; and Sioban Nelson, Anne Marie Rafferty, and Carol

Helmstadter, "Navigating the Political Straits in the Crimean War," in their *Notes on Nightingale: The Influence and Legacy of a Nursing Icon* (Ithaca, NY: ILR Press, 2010), chap. 2, 28–54.

49   without explicit medical orders for food: Nelson, Rafferty, and Helmstadter, "Navigating the Political Straits in the Crimean War," 35. Helmstadter, *Beyond Nightingale*, 115.

49   shocked by Nightingale's dictatorial style: Nelson, Rafferty, and Helmstadter, "Navigating the Political Straits in the Crimean War," 35.

49   "We do not look for many comforts": Helmstadter, "Nightingale's Team of Nurses," 65.

50   "'Thank you, ma'am'": Unless otherwise noted, all quotes and details about Seacole in this chapter are from her autobiography, *Wonderful Adventures of Mrs Seacole in Many Lands*.

51   a key, defining feature of nursing and of patient-centered care: Devon Brameier, Conor Hennessy, and Elisha Ngetich, "Mary Jane Seacole: The Shrouded Beacon of Patient-Centred Care," *Journal of the Nuffield Department of Surgical Sciences* 2, no. 2 (2021): doi.org/10.37707/jnds .v2i2.150.

52   hardly better than a brothel: Jane Robinson, "Age and Consequence," in her *The Charismatic Black Nurse Who Became a Heroine of the Crimea*, chap. 11, 190–91.

52   the *Morning Advertiser*: Robinson, "Age and Consequence," 143.

53   "testify to the worth of those services": Seacole and Salih, *Wonderful Adventures of Mrs Seacole in Many Lands*, appendix, 174.

53   in 1954, the Nurses Association of Jamaica named its headquarters: "Mary Seacole (1805–1881)," National Library of Jamaica, August 6, 2017, https://nlj.gov.jm/project/mary-seacole-1805-1881/.

53   Much later, after World War II: Feargus O'Sullivan and Brentin Mock, "U.K. Told Immigrants 'Go Home,' but Now It Needs Them," Bloomberg, April 21, 2020, www.bloomberg.com/news/articles/2020-04-21/the -u-k-is-failing-minority-health-care-workers.

53   it emerged that the government had destroyed landing cards: Nadine White, "The Government Is Asking Retired Windrush Nurses to Rejoin the NHS. Here's How They Feel," *HuffPost UK*, June 22, 2020, www.huffingtonpost.co.uk/entry/windrush-nurses-nhs-coronavirus_ uk_5e8351a4c5b603fbdf49ddf5; and Jack Guy, "Who Are the Windrush Generation? A British Scandal Explained," CNN, June 22, 2020,

www.cnn.com/2020/06/22/uk/windrush-explainer-cnn-poll-scli-intl
-gbr/index.html.

54   the status of being a British nurse was conditional: Gemma Mitchell,
       "Windrush Day: Nurses Demand Action on Racism and Inequality,"
       Nursing Times, June 22, 2020, www.nursingtimes.net/news/history-of
       -nursing/windrush-day-nurses-demand-action-on-racism-and-inequal
       ity-22-06-2020/.

54   a bizarre level of resistance: Amy Fleming, "Sculptor Defends His Mary
       Seacole Statue: 'If She Was White, Would There Be This Resistance?,'" The
       Guardian, June 21, 2016, www.theguardian.com/artanddesign/2016
       /jun/21/sculptor-defends-his-mary-seacole-statue-if-she-was-white
       -would-there-be-this-resistance.

54   a visible tattoo or natural Black hair: Georgina Cox, "Time for Nurs-
       ing to Eradicate Hair Discrimination," Journal of Clinical Nursing 30,
       no. 9–10 (2021): doi.org/10.1111/jocn.15708.

54   what the cost has been: Patricia D'Antonio, "What Do We Do about Flor-
       ence Nightingale?" Nursing Inquiry 29, no. 1 (2022): doi.org/10.1111
       /nin.12450.

54   history of nursing is far richer and more complicated: Anna Valdez,
       "Leading Change in the International Year of the Nurse and Midwife,"
       Teaching and Learning in Nursing 15, no. 2 (2020): doi.org/10.1016
       /j.teln.2020.01.003.

54   Nightingale lone-hero myth: Kylie Smith, "Moving Beyond Florence:
       Why We Need to Decolonize Nursing History," Nursing Clio, Janu-
       ary 23, 2022, nursingclio.org/2021/02/04/moving-beyond-florence
       -why-we-need-to-decolonize-nursing-history/.

55   "It was the class-structured British model": Helmstadter, Beyond Night-
       ingale, conclusion.

55   system of soldier "stewards" (nurses) assigned to hospital duty: Cha-
       rissa J. Threat, "The Politics of Intimate Care," in her Nursing Civil
       Rights: Gender and Race in the Army Nurse Corps, chap. 1, 12–19.

55   wanted to join up to nurse: Jane E. Schultz, "Women at the Front," in her
       Women at the Front: Hospital Workers in Civil War America (Chapel
       Hill: University of North Carolina Press, 2004), chap. 1, 12–44.

55   only to find she had already left: Thomas J. Brown, "The American In-
       vader," in his Dorothea Dix: New England Reformer (Cambridge, MA:
       Harvard University Press, 1998), chap. 10, 233.

56   the government would later offer wages to some: Details on Dix's crite-
      ria in this paragraph are from Thomas J. Brown, "A Huge Wild Beast Has
      Consumed my Life," in his *Dorothea Dix*, chap. 13, 280–323.

56   she did not meet the age requirement: Brown, "A Huge Wild Beast
      Has Consumed my Life," 304.

56   Dix hired about three thousand nurses: Schultz, "Women at the
      Front," 15.

56   started nursing by simply showing up: Alcott and Barton details are
      from Judith Giesberg, "Ms. Dix Comes to Washington," *New York
      Times*, April 27, 2011, archive.nytimes.com/opinionator.blogs.nytimes
      .com/2011/04/27/ms-dix-comes-to-washington/.

56   750,000 soldiers would be killed: Guy Gugliotta, "New Estimate Raises
      Civil War Death Toll," *New York Times*, April 2, 2012, www.nytimes
      .com/2012/04/03/science/civil-war-toll-up-by-20-percent-in-new
      -estimate.html.

56   2.5 percent of the total American population: "The Civil War by the
      Numbers," PBS, n.d., www.pbs.org/wgbh/americanexperience/features
      /death-numbers/.

56   more than half a million wounded: "Civil War Casualties," American
      Battlefield Trust, August 24, 2021, www.battlefields.org/learn/articles
      /civil-war-casualties.

57   After the carnage of Gettysburg: Schultz, "Women at the Front," 15.

57   Henry Martin: I first became aware of Henry Martin through a beauti-
      ful poem called "Bellringer," in the book *Playlist for the Apocalypse*, by
      Rita Dove.

57   "the soldiers that I seen laying on the floor": "The Life of Henry Martin,
      Bell Ringer for the University," *Virginia Magazine*, January 12, 2012,
      uvamagazine.org/videos/the_life_of_henry_martin_bell_ringer_for
      _the_university.

57   Black women especially struggled to get paid at all: Schultz, "Women at
      the Front," 41.

58   to wounded and dying soldiers: Martin G. Murray, "Traveling with the
      Wounded: Walt Whitman and Washington's Civil War Hospitals," Walt
      Whitman Archive, whitmanarchive.org/criticism/current/anc.00156.html.

58   "perhaps a thousand, and occasionally more still": Walt Whitman, "The
      Great Washington Hospitals," n.d., Walt Whitman Archive, whitman
      archive.org/published/periodical/journalism/tei/per.00210.html.

58   nightmares and flashbacks for the rest of his life: David Hsu, "Walt
      Whitman: An American Civil War Nurse Who Witnessed the Advent of
      Modern American Medicine," *Archives of Environmental and Occupa-
      tional Health* 65, no. 4 (2010): 238–39, doi.org/10.1080/19338244.2010
      .524510.

58   thirty dollars a month for hospital duty: Threat, "The Politics of Inti-
      mate Care," 17.

58   Some accounts: Jane E. Schultz, "Adjusting to Hospital Life," in her *Wom-
      en at the Front*, chap. 3, 88; and Murray, "Traveling with the Wounded."

59   taught soldiers to read and write in her off-hours: All details about Tay-
      lor are from Susie King Taylor, *Reminiscences of My Life in Camp with
      the 33d United States Colored Troops: Late 1st S.C. Volunteers* (self-pub.,
      1902), docsouth.unc.edu/neh/taylorsu/taylorsu.html; and from Eliza-
      beth Lindqwister, Karen Chittenden, and Micah Messenheimer, "Susie
      King Taylor: An African American Nurse and Teacher in the Civil War,"
      Library of Congress, 2019, www.loc.gov/ghe/cascade/index.html?appid
      =5be2377c246c4b5483e32ddd51d32dc0&bookmark=At%20War.

59   petitioning for one for years: Katherine Larson, *Bound for the Promised
      Land: Portrait of an American Hero* (New York: Ballantine Books, 2004),
      279.

60   first Black nurse to graduate from an American nursing school: Sarah
      Fielding, "Overlooked No More: Mary Eliza Mahoney, Who Opened
      Doors in Nursing," *New York Times*, February 19, 2022, www.nytimes
      .com/2022/02/19/obituaries/mary-eliza-mahoney-overlooked.html.

60   as their non-Black counterparts: M. Keaton Staupers, "Integration into
      the Military Service," in *No Time for Prejudice* (New York: Macmillan,
      1961), 120–21.

60   who served throughout the war: For details in this paragraph, see Dar-
      lene Clark Hine, "Racism, Status, and the Professionalization of Black
      Nursing," in her *Black Women in White*, chap. 5, 102–3.

61   was included in the army: Darlene Clark Hine, "'We Shall Not Be Left
      Out': World War II and the Integration of Nursing," in her *Black Women
      in White*, chap. 8, 162–86.

61   nine thousand Black graduate nurses: Staupers, "Integration into the
      Military Service," 118.

61   "committed to a policy of discrimination," she said: For this and details
      in the previous paragraph, see Hine, "'We Shall Not Be Left Out,'" 162–86.

62 before he was transferred to the white hospital: "Interview Transcript: Prudence Burns Burrell," Veterans History Project, Library of Congress, n.d., memory.loc.gov/diglib/vhp-stories/loc.natlib.afc2001001.04747 /transcript?ID=sr0001.

62 "'as another example of discrimination'": Pia Marie Winters Jordan, author phone interview.

62 Tuskegee Air Force Base: Pia Winters Jordan, "Louise Lomax," Tuskegee Army Nurses, n.d., www.tuskegeearmynurses.info/2019/06/25/louise -lomax/.

63 a 1942 *New York Times* headline proclaimed: "Need Emphasized for More Nurses; Growing Shortage in Hospitals Discussed at Meeting of Recruitment Group Women Urged to Enroll 20,000 Students Must Be Added to Mid-Term Lists in Schools, Unit Hears," *New York Times*, September 23, 1942, www.nytimes.com/1942/09/23/archives/need-empha sized-for-more-nurses-growing-shortage-in-hospitals.html?search ResultPosition=1.

63 earn you a dishonorable discharge: Hine, "'We Shall Not Be Left Out,'" 174.

63 found himself filling potholes in India: O'Lynn and Tranbarger, "History of Men in Nursing," 27.

63 but were being barred: Charissa J. Threat, "Nurse or Soldier?" in her *Nursing Civil Rights*, chap. 3, 75.

63 In 1943, the army raised its quota: Details and numbers in this paragraph are from Charissa J. Threat, "The Negro Nurse—A Citizen Fighting for Democracy," in her *Nursing Civil Rights*, chap. 2, 45–47.

64 back-channel campaign to remove the restrictions: Staupers, "Integration into the Military Services," 116–17.

64 provide adequate care for its soldiers: Hine, "'We Shall Not Be Left Out,'" 162–86.

65 Black nurses would now be accepted: Staupers, "Integration into the Military Services," 116–17.

65 a right to care for their countrymen: Analysis here and throughout this chapter is from Threat author interview.

65 "from the full realization of their civil rights": Hine, "'We Shall Not Be Left Out,'" 181.

65 "You would think I was being born again": All quotes from and details

about Leftenant-Colon are from Nancy Leftenant-Colon in-person author interview, June 22, 2021.

66   military accepted male nurses: Charissa J. Threat, "An American Challenge," in her *Nursing Civil Rights*, chap. 4, 104–5.

66   "Nursing is focused on the health of the individual and the community": Threat phone interview with the author.

CHAPTER 4: COMMUNITY

67   handbook everyone carried with them: All details about and quotes from the Wickhams throughout this chapter are from in-person interviews with the Wickhams and in-person observation of the diabetes seminar, March 24, 2022.

67   Stephen Wickham, RN: I first heard about the Wickhams' diabetes program from Blake Farmer, "2 Nurses in Tennessee Preach 'Diabetes Reversal,'" NPR, July 22, 2019, www.npr.org/sections/health -shots/2019/07/22/733748382/2-nurses-in-tennessee-preach-diabetes -reversal.

68   "undoes everything the sugar's been doing": Wickham attributes this idea to Robert Lustig, MD.

69   a more resistant starch: Christine McKinney, "What Is Resistant Starch?" The Johns Hopkins Patient Guide to Diabetes, December 2, 2020, hop kinsdiabetesinfo.org/what-is-resistant-starch/.

69   small community: Dan Buettner, "Loma Linda, California," Blue Zones, May 4, 2021, www.bluezones.com/exploration/loma-linda-california/.

70   has been shown in randomized controlled trials: *Nurse-Family Partnership Fact Research Trials and Outcomes*, PDF, n.d., www.nursefam ilypartnership.org/wp-content/uploads/2022/03/NFP-Research-Trials -and-Outcomes.pdf.

71   Some existing studies: Sarah J. Hallberg, "Reversing Type 2 Diabetes: A Narrative Review of the Evidence," *Nutrients* 11, no. 4 (2019): 766, doi .org/10.3390/nu11040766.

71   diabetes remission: "International Experts Outline Diabetes Remission Diagnosis Criteria," Press Release, American Diabetes Association, August 30, 2021, www.diabetes.org/newsroom/press-releases/2021/inter national-experts-outline-diabetes-remission-diagnosis-criteria.

72   Diabetes is the most expensive chronic disease: National Center for

Chronic Disease Prevention and Health Promotion, "Cost-Effectiveness of Diabetes Interventions," Centers for Disease Control and Prevention, March 7, 2022, www.cdc.gov/chronicdisease/programs-impact/pop /diabetes.htm#:~:text=Diabetes%20is%20the%20most%20expensive %20chronic%20condition%20in%20our%20nation.&text=%241%20 out%20of%20every%20%244,caring%20for%20people%20with%20di abetes.&text=%24237%20billion%E2%80%A1(c)%20is,(c)%20on%20 reduced%20productivity.

72   Diabetes outcomes are only worsening: "Major Study of Diabetes Trends Shows Americans' Blood Sugar Control Is Getting Worse," Johns Hopkins Bloomberg School of Public Health, n.d., publichealth .jhu.edu/2021/major-study-of-diabetes-trends-shows-americans-blood -sugar-control-is-getting-worse.

72   over 96 percent white: "QuickFacts: Polk County, Tennessee," United States Census Bureau, n.d., www.census.gov/quickfacts/polkcounty tennessee.

72   a large majority is observantly Christian: "Religion in Polk County, Tennessee," Best Places, n.d., www.bestplaces.net/religion/county/tennes see/polk.

72   15 percent of the population has diabetes: "Profiles of Health in Tennessee Polk County," Sycamore Institute, n.d., www.sycamoreinstitutetn .org/wp-content/uploads/2018/07/Polk-Co-Tennessee-County-Health -Profile-July-2018.pdf.

72   10 percent in the United States on average: "The Facts, Stats, and Impacts of Diabetes," Centers for Disease Control and Prevention, n.d., www .cdc.gov/diabetes/library/spotlights/diabetes-facts-stats.html#:~:text =Key%20findings%20include%3A,t%20know%20they%20have% 20it.

73   nearly two thousand people die of diabetes each year: "Stats of the State of Tennessee," Centers for Disease Control and Prevention, 2017, www .cdc.gov/nchs/pressroom/states/tennessee/tennessee.htm.

73   Most Americans consume only about ten grams a day: Katherine McManus, "Should I Be Eating More Fiber?" *Harvard Health Blog*, February 27, 2019, www.health.harvard.edu/blog/should-i-be-eating-more -fiber-2019022115927.

73   by eating, for instance: "Chart of High-Fiber Foods" Mayo Clinic, Mayo Foundation for Medical Education and Research, January 5, 2021,

www.mayoclinic.org/healthy-lifestyle/nutrition-and-healthy-eating/in
-depth/high-fiber-foods/art-20050948.

73 decreasing blood sugar spikes: "Fiber: The Carb That Helps You Manage Diabetes," Centers for Disease Control and Prevention, February 4,
2022, www.cdc.gov/diabetes/library/features/role-of-fiber.html.

73 Lee Kent: All quotes from and details about Lee Kent are from two author phone interviews, January 13, 2020, and July 20, 2022.

75 three hundred dollars a vial: S. Vincent Rajkumar, "The High Cost of
Insulin in the United States: An Urgent Call to Action," *Mayo Clinic Proceedings* 95, no. 1 (2020): 22–28, doi.org/10.1016/j.mayocp.2019.11.013.

75 public health nursing and community health nursing overlap: "Public Health Nursing," American Nurses Association, n.d., www.nursing
world.org/practice-policy/workforce/public-health-nursing/.

76 the ripple effects would change the world: "Baptism of Fire: Henry
Street Settlement," video, Henry Street Settlement, September 21, 2018,
www.henrystreet.org/about/our-history/exhibit-the-house-on-henry
-street/baptism-video/.

76 Wald had recently graduated: Unless otherwise noted, all information
about Wald and her work and quotes from Wald in this chapter are
from her autobiography, Lillian D. Wald, *The House on Henry Street*
(New York: Henry Holt and Company, 1915).

77 the family couldn't pay: "Baptism of Fire: Henry Street Settlement."

77 English-French Boarding and Day School for Young Ladies: "Lillian D.
Wald (1867–1940)—Nurse, Social Worker, Women's Rights Activist and
Founder of Henry Street Settlement," Social Welfare History Project,
Virginia Commonwealth University, n.d., socialwelfare.library.vcu.edu
/people/wald-lillian/.

79 particular moment in the history of the Lower East Side: Details about
the Lower East Side in this paragraph are from in-person author visit
to *Henry Street Settlement* exhibit and from an interview with Henry
Street public historian Katie Vogel, April 4, 2022.

79 Twenty-seven percent of babies: John S. Billings, "Vital Statistics of
New York City and Brooklyn: Six Years Ending May 31, 1890," Department of the Interior, U.S. Census Office, 1894.

80 Wald had romantic relationships with two of the women: "Lillian Wald,"
Henry Street Settlement, n.d., www.henrystreet.org/about/our-history
/lillian-wald/.

80   on-site clinic: Details in this paragraph are from in-person author visit to *Henry Street Settlement* exhibit and from Vogel author interview.

81   "and independence of patients.": Wald, The *House on Henry Street*, 27.

81   "of professional etiquette.": Wald, *The House on Henry Street*, 33–34.

81   paying them all the same wage: Hine, "Racism, Status, and the Profes-sionalization of Black Nursing," 101.

82   Edith Carter, Emma Wilson, and other Black nurses: For general infor-mation about Tyler and her colleagues, see Mary Elizabeth Carnegie, "Stony the Road," in *The Path We Tread: Blacks in Nursing Worldwide, 1854–1994* (Sudbury, MA: Jones and Bartlett Publishers, 2000), chap. 5, 155–56.

82   Stillman House would eventually provide: Rhonda Evans, "San Juan Hill and the Black Nurses of the Stillman Settlement," New York Public Library, January 16, 2020, www.nypl.org/blog/2019/12/01/san-juan-hill -black-nurses-stillman-settlement.

82   *New York Times* covered Wald's nurses: "Unique Settlement on Henry Street: In This District the Sick Are Given All Necessary Care and Proper Nursing at Their Homes Instead of Going to Hospital," *New York Times*, July 21, 1907.

83   two hundred thousand visits each year: Statistics from "Lillian Wald."

83   about 10 percent: Wald, *The House on Henry Street*, 42.

83   at one hospital, it was 51 percent: All statistics by Wald, *The House on Henry Street*, 38.

84   She said children's play was a matter of "dignity": Wald, *The House on Henry Street*, 95.

84   led the city to adopt the idea in 1902: "Lillian Wald."

84   within the purview of nursing: In-person author visit to *Henry Street Settlement* exhibit and author interview with Vogel.

84   at the very center of what she did: Helena Huntington Smith, "Profiles: Rampant but Respectable," *The New Yorker*, December 14, 1929.

85   at the age of seventy-three: "Lillian Wald Dies: Friend of the Poor," *New York Times*, September 2, 1940.

85   WE ARE HERE TO HELP!: In-person author visit to *Henry Street Settlement* exhibit and author interview with Vogel.

87   so the company ended the program: Information in this and the pre-vious paragraph is from Karen Buhler-Wilkerson, *No Place like Home:*

A History of Nursing and Home Care in the United States (Baltimore, MD: Johns Hopkins University Press, 2003), 163–64.

87   roughly 60 percent: U.S. Bureau of Labor Statistics, "Registered Nurses."

87   even at Walmart: "Locate the Services Available in Your Area," Walmart Health, n.d., www.walmart.com/cp/care-clinics/1224932.

87   people experiencing homelessness: "Library Nurse Program," Pima County, n.d., webcms.pima.gov/cms/one.aspx?portalId=169&pageId=39186.

88   something was going very wrong: Unless otherwise noted, all information about the measles outbreak and quotes by and about Ash are from author phone interview with Tobi Ash, January 18, 2022.

88   as much as two hours later: "Top Things Parents Need to Know About Measles," Centers for Disease Control and Prevention, November 5, 2020, www.cdc.gov/measles/about/parents-top4.html#:~:text=Your%20child%20can%20get%20measles,rash%20through%20four%20days%20afterward.

90   thought that pediatricians were exceedingly rich: Amanda Schaffer, "Amid a Measles Outbreak, an Ultra-Orthodox Nurse Fights Vaccination Fears in Her Community," *The New Yorker*, January 25, 2019, www.newyorker.com/news/as-told-to/amid-a-measles-outbreak-an-ultra-orthodox-nurse-fights-vaccination-fears-in-her-community.

90   1,282 cases of measles resulted from the outbreak: Centers for Disease Control and Prevention, "National Update on Measles Cases and Outbreaks—United States, January 1–October 1, 2019," *Morbidity and Mortality Weekly Report*, CDC, October 10, 2019, www.cdc.gov/mmwr/volumes/68/wr/mm6840e2.htm.

CHAPTER 5: ENDINGS

92   Mariana Sandarovscaia, RN: All quotes from Sarah Creed, Mariana Sandarovscaia, "Ahmad," and Tim Boon and all information about Good Shepherd and the hospice work described are from an in-person author visit to Good Shepherd and in-person interviews with Mariana Sandarovscaia, Sarah Creed, "Ahmad," and Tim Boon, January 12 and 13, 2022.

100   despite the disapproval of her family: Caroline Richmond, "Dame Cicely Saunders, Founder of the Modern Hospice Movement, Dies," *The BMJ*, n.d., www.bmj.com/content/suppl/2005/07/18/331.7509.DC1.

100 "invalided out" of nursing: Unless otherwise noted, biographical details and information about Saunders's work throughout this section
are from Cicely M. Saunders and David Clark, *Cicely Saunders: Selected
Writings 1958–2004* (Oxford, UK: Oxford University Press, 2012), xiii–
xxviii.

100 David Tasma: For photograph of and information on Tasma, see Chris
Olver, "Short Biography of Dame Cecily Saunders (1918–2005)." Ar-
chives of Dame Cicely Saunders (1918–2005): Cataloguing the Papers
of the Modern Hospice Pioneer, n.d., cicelysaundersarchive.wordpress
.com/tag/david-tasma/.

100 What we know of Tasma's life is harrowing: Yasmin Gunaratnam, "Eros,"
in her *Death and the Migrant: Bodies, Borders, and Care* (London:
Bloomsbury Academic, 2015), chap. 2.

101 without being able to say goodbye: Richmond, "Dame Cicely Saunders,
Founder of the Modern Hospice Movement, Dies."

101 desertion of the dying: Olver, "Short Biography of Dame Cicely Saunders."

101 open to those of all faiths or none: "Dame Cicely Saunders: Her Life and
Work," St Christopher's Hospice, July 8, 2020, www.stchristophers.org
.uk/about/damecicelysaunders.

101 Camillus de Lellis: O'Lynn and Tranbarger, "History of Men in Nursing," 20–21.

102 she said in a speech in 1981: Cicely M. Saunders and David Clark, "Tem-
pleton Prize Speech," in *Cicely Saunders: Selected Writings, 1958–2004*
(Oxford, UK: Oxford University Press, 2012), 58.

102 "live until you die": "Cicely Saunders," Oxford Essential Quotations.
n.d., www.oxfordreference.com/view/10.1093/acref/9780191826719
.001.0001/q-oro-ed4-00009140.

102 in 1963: Stephen R. Connor, "Development of Hospice and Palliative
Care in the United States," *OMEGA: Journal of Death and Dying* 56,
no. 1 (2008): 90, doi.org/10.2190/om.56.1.h.

103 "She made an indelible impression": Patricia Sullivan, "Obituary: Florence Wald, 91; Started Hospice Movement in US," *Boston Globe*, November 14, 2008, archive.boston.com/bostonglobe/obituaries/articles
/2008/11/14/florence_wald_91_started_hospice_movement_in_us/.

103 first hospice organization in Massachusetts: "History and Mission," Good
Shepherd Community Care, n.d., gscommunitycare.org/History-Mission.

103 all the costs for the terminal illness: Office of the Assistant Secretary for Planning and Evaluation, "Medicare's Hospice Benefit: Revising the Payment System to Better Reflect Visit Intensity," U.S. Department of Health and Human Services, n.d., aspe.hhs.gov/reports/medicares -hospice-benefit-revising-payment-system-better-reflect-visit-intensity -0#:~:text=The%20Medicare%20hospice%20benefit%20was,illness %20runs%20its%20normal%20course.

103 doesn't mean they go without medical care: "What Are Palliative Care and Hospice Care?" National Institute on Aging, U.S. Department of Health and Human Services, May 14, 2021, www.nia.nih.gov/health /what-are-palliative-care-and-hospice-care.

103 can be continued as usual: Centers for Medicare and Medicaid Services, "Medicare Hospice Benefits," Medicare.gov, n.d., www.medicare .gov/Pubs/pdf/02154-Medicare-Hospice-Benefits.PDF.

104 hospice facilities: Sam Halabi, "Selling Hospice," *Journal of Law, Medicine and Ethics* 42, no. 4 (2014): 442–54, doi.org/10.1111/jlme.12167.

105 Rodney Mesquias: Jerry Soucy, RN, first told me about this case.

105 twenty years in prison for fraud and money laundering: U.S. Attorney's Office, Southern District of Texas, "Owner of Texas Chain of Hospice Companies Sentenced for $150 Million Health Care Fraud and Money Laundering Scheme," Press Release, Justic.gov, December 16, 2020, www.justice.gov/usao-sdtx/pr/owner-texas-chain-hospice-companies -sentenced-150-million-health-care-fraud-and-money.

108 Ward 5B: I first heard about 5B through the podcast *See You Now* with Shawna Butler.

108 San Francisco General Hospital: Unless otherwise noted, all information about Ward 5B in this section is from the documentary *5B*, directed by Dan Krauss (RYOT, 2018), 5bfilm.com/.

109 Jerry Soucy: All quotes and information about Soucy throughout this chapter are from an author telephone interview with Jerry Soucy, December 8, 2021.

CHAPTER 6: AUTONOMY

113 In February 1935: Rose Holz, "Nurse Gordon on Trial: Those Early Days of the Birth Control Clinic Movement Reconsidered," *Journal of Social History* 39, no. 1 (2005): 112–40, doi.org/10.1353/jsh.2005.0106.

113 free lecture on birth control later that month: "Women Crowd Birth

Control Trial: State Agents Tell of Visits to Clinic Here," *The Milwaukee Journal*, April 3, 1935, 32.

114 sentenced to six months in prison: "Birth Control 'Sales' Denied: Supplies Given 'Free' for a Fee, Is Defense in Woman's Trial Here," *Milwaukee Journal*, April 4, 1935, 9.

114 posted $750 bail: "Posts Bond," *Milwaukee Sentinel*, March 6, 1935, 4.

114 She and her supporters wrote to newspapers: Holz, "Nurse Gordon on Trial," 124.

114 giving away the diaphragms for free: "Birth Control 'Sales' Denied," 9.

114 The jury selection was contentious: "Jury Chosen to Try Birth Control Case," *Milwaukee Sentinel*, April 2, 1935, 9.

115 stop turning the trial into a lecture on birth control: "Birth Control 'Sales' Denied," 9.

115 "That is hearsay and highly prejudicial": "Adele Gordon Airs Views on Birth Control: Defendant Insists Her Work Is a Boon to Race," *Milwaukee Sentinel*, April 4, 1935, 13.

115 some women in the courthouse openly wept: "Birth Control Jury Frees Woman Here," *Milwaukee Journal*, April 4, 1935, 44.

115 The jury deliberated for just twenty-five minutes: Holz, "Nurse Gordon on Trial," 126.

115 free birth control lectures and clinic, open once more: "Free Lecture 'Birth Control' Instructive, Educational, Scientific," *Milwaukee Journal*, May 10, 1935, 21.

116 Some nurses and midwives argue: Meghan Eagen Torkko and Susan Yanow, "The Critical Role of Midwives in Safe Self Managed Abortion," *Journal of Midwifery and Women's Health* 66, no. 6 (2021): 795–800, doi.org/10.1111/jmwh.13289.

117 from antiquity onward: Norman Himes, "Medical History of Contraception," *New England Journal of Medicine* 210 (March 1934):DOI: 10.1056/NEJM193403152101103.

117 chewed cotton root as a contraceptive or abortifacient: "Reproduction and Resistance Hidden Voices: Enslaved Women in the Lowcountry and U.S. South," Lowcountry Digital History Initiative, College of Charleston, n.d., ldhi.library.cofc.edu/exhibits/show/hidden-voices/resisting-enslavement/reproduction-and-resistance.

117 Mexican women chewed the root of a wild yam: Crystal Raypole, "The History of Birth Control: Early Methods, Legal Issues, & More," Health-

line. Healthline Media, June 28, 2021, https://www.healthline.com/health/birth-control/history-of-birth-control#modern-methods.

117   or to induce abortion: For instance, Hildegard von Bingen includes remedies to bring about menstruation. Hildegard von Bingen, trans. Priscilla Throop, *Causes and Cures: The Complete English Translation of Hildegardis Causae et Curae Libri VI* (Charlotte, VT: MedievalMS, 2008), 149.

117   through the mid-1800s: "Abortion: Solidly Rooted in America's History," Planned Parenthood, n.d., www.plannedparenthoodaction.org/issues/abortion/abortion-central-history-reproductive-health-care-america; and "Anthony Comstock's 'Chastity' Laws," PBS, www.pbs.org/wgbh/americanexperience/features/pill-anthony-comstocks-chastity-laws/.

117   In the 1850s: Ellen Chesler, "Seeds of Rebellion," in her *Woman of Valor: Margaret Sanger and the Birth Control Movement in America* (New York: Simon and Schuster Paperbacks, 2007), chap. 3, 63.

117   by the 1880s, all states had laws restricting: "Historical Abortion Law Timeline: 1850 to Today," Planned Parenthood Action Fund, n.d., www.plannedparenthoodaction.org/issues/abortion/abortion-central-history-reproductive-health-care-america/historical-abortion-law-timeline-1850-today.

118   outlawed the distribution of information about it: Margaret Sanger, *The Autobiography of Margaret Sanger* (New York: W. W. Norton, 1938), 210–23.

118   Sanger remembered her mother's life: Ellen Chesler, "Ghosts," in her *Woman of Valor,* chap. 1, 40–41.

118   wanted to be a physician so she could help her mother: Sanger, "Books Are the Compasses," in her *Autobiography of Margaret Sanger,* chap. 3, 45.

118   Then, in 1910: Michelle Goldberg, "Awakenings: On Margaret Sanger," *The Nation,* June 29, 2015, www.thenation.com/article/archive/awakenings-margaret-sanger/.

118   In her autobiography, Sanger wrote: Sanger, "The Turbid Ebb and Flow of Misery," in her *Autobiography of Margaret Sanger,* chap. 7, 89.

119   about one-third of women: Chesler, "Seeds of Rebellion," 64.

119   many ways women attempted to induce abortion: Sanger, *Autobiography of Margaret Sanger,* 89.

119 "I knew I could no longer go back": Sanger, *Autobiography of Margaret Sanger*, 92.

120 The push to criminalize abortion: Dine, "Scarlet Letters."

120 the work of the newly formed American Medical Association: Ramtin Arablouei and Rund Abdelfatah, "Abortion Was Once Common Practice in America. A Small Group of Doctors Changed That," NPR, June 6, 2022, www.npr.org/2022/06/06/1103372543/abortion-was-once-common-practice-in-america-a-small-group-of-doctors-changed-th. Context on the AMA's opposition to abortion also found in Chesler, *Woman of Valor*, 64.

120 a matter of business competition: Erin Blakemore, "The Criminalization of Abortion Began as a Business Tactic," History.com, January 22, 2018, www.history.com/news/the-criminalization-of-abortion-began-as-a-business-tactic.

120 as did other practitioners: Leslie J. Reagan, "Linking Midwives and Abortion in the Progressive Era," *Bulletin of the History of Medicine* 69, no. 4 (1995): 569–98.

120 birth rates were declining among U.S.-born white women: Michael R. Haines, "American Fertility in Transition: New Estimates of Birth Rates in the United States, 1900–1910," *Demography* 26, no. 1 (1989): 137–48, doi.org/10.2307/2061500.

120 "willful sterility" was an unforgiveable sin: Dorothy E. Roberts, "The Dark Side of Birth Control," in her *Killing the Black Body*, chap. 2, 57–62.

120 characterized by quantity, not quality: Linda Gordon, "Professionalization," in her *The Moral Property of Women: A History of Birth Control Politics in America* (Urbana and Chicago: University of Illinois Press, 2007), chap. 9, 180.

120 federally funded program of forced sterilization: Lisa Ko, "Unwanted Sterilization and Eugenics Programs in the United States," *Independent Lens*, PBS, November 19, 2020, www.pbs.org/independentlens/blog/unwanted-sterilization-and-eugenics-programs-in-the-united-states/.

121 passing down recipes and devices for contraception for generations: Sanger, *Autobiography of Margaret Sanger*, 93–105.

121 In Connecticut, for instance: Margaret Sanger, "The Status of Birth Control: 1938," *The New Republic*, July 23, 2022, newrepublic.com/article/100850/the-status-birth-control-1938.

121 wait until women had the vote to act on birth control: Sanger, *Autobiography of Margaret Sanger*, 93.

121 the poor had a sacred right to bread: Cynthia Anne Connolly, "'I Am a Trained Nurse': The Nursing Identity of Anarchist and Radical Emma Goldman," *Nursing History Review* 18, no. 1 (2010): 84–99, doi.org /10.1891/1062–8061.18.84.

121 She loved the work: Emma Goldman, *Living My Life: Both Volumes, Complete and Unabridged* (Pantianos Classics, 2018), 1:94–95.

122 she didn't have good information: Goldman, *Living My Life*, 1:127–28.

122 She was arrested for violating: "Today in History—Emma Goldman," Library of Congress, n.d., www.loc.gov/item/today-in-history/february -11/.

122 Later, the two women became estranged: Chesler, *Woman of Valor*, 86–87.

122 also used to prevent uterine prolapse: Chesler, *Woman of Valor*, 150–53.

123 it had served 464 women: Chesler, *Woman of Valor*, 151–53.

123 which had previously been illegal: Chesler, *Woman of Valor*, 159– 60.

123 She famously spoke to the women of the Ku Klux Klan: Alexis McGill Johnson, "I'm the Head of Planned Parenthood. We're Done Making Excuses for Our Founder," *New York Times*, April 17, 2021, www .nytimes.com/2021/04/17/opinion/planned-parenthood-margaret -sanger.html.

123 harnessed the birth control movement to eugenic ideas: Michelle Goldberg, writing in *The Nation*, described Sanger's use of the ideology this way: "Eugenics offered respectability to a cause seen as scandalous and marginal." Goldberg, "Awakenings: On Margaret Sanger."

124 argue that birth control and abortion are a kind of genocide: "Opposition Claims about Margaret Sanger–Planned Parenthood," Planned Parenthood, n.d., www.plannedparenthood.org/uploads/filer_public /cc/2e/cc2e84f2-126f-41a5-a24b-43e093c47b2c/210414-sanger-oppo sition-claims-p01.pdf.

124 forced upon Black communities: Writing in Rewire, journalist Imani Gandy shed light on this: "Sanger was passionate about contraception— perhaps to a fault—and her fervor about promoting her birth control agenda led her to align herself with eugenicists, along with racists and an assortment of people of questionable character. But it is simply

untrue that Margaret Sanger wanted to exterminate the Black race. This is a flat-out lie." Imani Gandy, "How False Narratives of Margaret Sanger Are Being Used to Shame Black Women," Rewire, August 20, 2015, rewirenewsgroup.com/2015/08/20/false-narratives-margaret-sanger-used-shame-black-women/.

124 to set up clinics in Black neighborhoods: Amita Kelly, "Fact Check: Was Planned Parenthood Started to 'Control' the Black Population?" NPR, August 14, 2015, www.npr.org/sections/itsallpolitics/2015/08/14/432080520/fact-check-was-planned-parenthood-started-to-control-the-black-population.

124 to reach people in rural areas: Jessie M. Rodrique, "The Black Community and the Birth Control Movement," from Dorothy O. Helly and Susan M. Reverby, eds., *Gendered Domains* (Ithaca, NY: Cornell University Press, 2018): 244–60, https://doi.org/10.7591/9781501720741–019.

124 instead predicated on a physician's autonomy: Jeffrey Toobin, "The People's Choice," *The New Yorker*, January 21, 2013, www.newyorker.com/magazine/2013/01/28/the-peoples-choice-2.

124 "should be terminated.": Roe V. Wade (https://supreme.justia.com/cases/federal/us/410/113/ January 22, 1973).

124 her embrace of eugenics: For deeper analysis of this, see Roberts, *Killing the Black Body*, 72–6.

125 Michelle Drew's midwifery practice: Unless otherwise noted, all quotes and information about Drew's work are from a Zoom interview with Michelle Drew, February 7, 2022.

127 she swallowed back tears: "Black Midwives: A History Forum," UVA School of Nursing, n.d., www.nursing.virginia.edu/nursing-history/events-cnhi/.

127 sought to sideline: Kennedy Austin, "End Racial Disparities in Maternal Health, Call a Midwife," February 2, 2020, www.publichealth.columbia.edu/public-health-now/news/end-racial-disparities-maternal-health-call-midwife.

127 and then eradicate them: "Black History Month: Honoring Black Grand Midwives and Supporting Black Midwives Today," Quickening: The News Site of the American College of Nurse-Midwives, February 18, 2021, quickening.midwife.org/roundtable/black-history-month-honoring-black-grand-midwives-and-supporting-black-midwives-today/.

127 only 6 percent of nurse midwives are Black: *American Midwifery Cer-*

tification Board 2020 Demographic Report, n.d., www.amcbmidwife
.org/docs/default-source/reports/demographic-report-2019.pdf?sfvrsn
=23f30668_2.

128 at up to twelve weeks' gestation: Claire Cain Miller and Margot Sanger-
Katz, "Medication Abortions Are Increasing: What They Are and Where
Women Get Them," *New York Times,* May 9, 2022, www.nytimes.com
/2022/05/09/upshot/abortion-pills-medication-roe-v-wade.html.

128 as a way of reducing access altogether: "The Availability and Use of
Medication Abortion," Kaiser Family Foundation, April 6, 2022, www
.kff.org/womens-health-policy/fact-sheet/the-availability-and-use-of
-medication-abortion/.

128 even facilitating access in U.S. states where it is illegal: A study of mail-
ordered pills found that the pills were legitimate and effective. Chloe
Murtagh et al., "Exploring the Feasibility of Obtaining Mifepristone and
Misoprostol from the Internet," *Contraception* 97, no. 4 (2018): 287–91,
doi.org/10.1016/j.contraception.2017.09.016.

128 The World Health Organization has reported: *Medical Management
of Abortion,* World Health Organization–Geneva, 2018, apps.who.int
/iris/bitstream/handle/10665/278968/9789241550406-eng.pdf?ua=1.

128 in the absence of any clinical care at all: Melissa Madera et al.,
"Experiences Seeking, Sourcing, and Using Abortion Pills at Home
in the United States Through an Online Telemedicine Service," *SSM–
Qualitative Research in Health* 2 (2022): 100075, doi.org/10.1016/j
.ssmqr.2022.100075; Julie Jenkins et al., "Abortion with Pills: Review of
Current Options in the United States," *Journal of Midwifery and Wom-
en's Health* 66, no. 6 (2021): 749–57, doi.org/10.1111/jmwh.13291.

128 certified nurse-midwife: All quotes by and information on Stephanie
from Hey Jane are from author phone interview, April 8, 2022.

130 Nurses for Sexual and Reproductive Health: Anna Brown, author phone
interview, April 27, 2022.

131 Monica McLemore, PhD, RN: McLemore author phone interview.

132 McLemore headed a study: Monica R. McLemore, Amy Levi, and E. Angel James, "Recruitment and Retention Strategies for Expert Nurses in
Abortion Care Provision," *Contraception* 91, no. 6 (2015): 474–79, doi
.org/10.1016/j.contraception.2015.02.007.

132 a framework developed by Black women: "RJ Founding Mothers," Black
Women for Reproductive Justice, August 8, 2012, bwrj.wordpress

.com/2012/08/08/151/; and Loretta Ross, "Understanding Reproductive Justice: Transforming the Pro-Choice Movement," *Off Our Backs* 36, no. 4 (2006): 14–19.

132 "I come from the tradition of Nurse-Family Partnership": Monica McLemore, "Re-imagining What's Possible: A Future Where Reproductive Justice Is Achieved," Barnard Center Free Lecture Series, Lecture Presented by the University of Washington, April 13, 2022.

133 One nurse practitioner whom I'll call Hannah.: Author telephone interview with "Hannah," March 14, 2022.

CHAPTER 7: ENVIRONMENT

136 their steps illuminated only by flashlights: Gail Deutsch, Marc Dorian, and Adam Sechrist, "Nurses Who Saved NICU Babies Remember Harrowing, Triumphant Hurricane Night," ABC News, November 3, 2012, abcnews.go.com/Health/nicu-nurses-saved-babies-remember-harrow ing-triumphant-hurricane/story?id=17632993; Elizabeth Cohen and Senior Medical Correspondent, "N.Y. Hospital Staff Carry Sick Babies Down 9 Flights of Stairs During Evacuation," CNN, October 31, 2012, www.cnn.com/2012/10/30/health/sandy-hospital/index.html.

136 phone service in the city cut in and out: Sharon Begley, "Sandy Exposed Hospitals' Lack of Disaster Preparedness," *Insurance Journal*, November 6, 2012, www.insurancejournal.com/news/national/2012 /11/06/269512.htm.

137 some of what nurses are already noticing: Katie Huffling phone interview with author, June 8, 2021.

137 killing tens of thousands of people: Jason Beaubien, "Whatever Happened to . . . the Mysterious Kidney Disease Striking Central America?" NPR, August 26, 2019, www.npr.org/sections/goatsandsoda/2019 /08/26/753834371/whatever-happened-to-the-mysterious-kidney -disease-striking-central-america; Catharina Wesseling et al., "Chronic Kidney Disease of Non-Traditional Origin in Mesoamerica: A Disease Primarily Driven by Occupational Heat Stress," *Revista Panamericana de Salud Pública* 44 (2020): 1, doi.org/10.26633/rpsp.2020.15; Sandra Peraza et al., "Decreased Kidney Function Among Agricultural Workers in El Salvador," *American Journal of Kidney Diseases* 59, no. 4 (2012): 531–40, doi.org/10.1053/j.ajkd.2011.11.039.

138 nearly a quarter of the population: Senaka Rajapakse, Mitrakrishnan
     Chrishan Shivanthan, and Mathu Selvarajah, "Chronic Kidney Disease
     of Unknown Etiology in Sri Lanka," *International Journal of Occupa-
     tional and Environmental Health* 22, no. 3 (2016): 259, doi.org/10.1080
     /10773525.2016.1203097.

138 popped up in other very hot regions: Cecilia Sorensen and Ramon
     Garcia-Trabanino, "A New Era of Climate Medicine—Addressing Heat-
     Triggered Renal Disease," *New England Journal of Medicine* 381, no. 8
     (2019):693–96, doi.org/10.1056/nejmp1907859. "We may have now
     reached a physiological limit, in terms of heat exposure, at which accli-
     matization and behavioral modifications can no longer overcome the
     biologic stressors of unsafe working conditions and environmental ex-
     posures in these hot spot communities."

138 parts of Africa and the Middle East: Moussa El Khayat et al., "Impacts
     of Climate Change and Heat Stress on Farmworkers' Health: A Scoping
     Review," *Frontiers in Public Health* 10 (2022): Figure 2, doi.org/10.3389
     /fpubh.2022.782811.

138 workers in high-altitude coffee-growing villages: Timothy S. Laux et al.,
     "Nicaragua Revisited: Evidence of Lower Prevalence of Chronic Kidney
     Disease in a High-Altitude, Coffee-Growing Village," *Journal of Nephrolo-
     gy* 25, no. 4 (2011): 533–40, https://www.ncbi.nlm.nih.gov/pmc/articles
     /PMC4405255/.

138 average global temperatures have risen by two degrees Fahrenheit:
     "World of Change," NASA, n.d., earthobservatory.nasa.gov/world-of
     -change.

138 10 percent more moisture in the air now: Matthew Cappucci, "Analysis:
     Increasing Humidity, Driven in Part by Climate Change, Is Making Even
     Modest Heat Waves Unbearable," *Washington Post*, August 13, 2019,
     www.washingtonpost.com/weather/2019/08/13/increasing-humidity
     -driven-part-by-climate-change-is-making-even-modest-heat-waves-un
     bearable/.

138 classified as heat stroke, which can be fatal: "Heatstroke," Mayo Clinic,
     n.d., www.mayoclinic.org/diseases-conditions/heat-stroke/symptoms
     -causes/syc-20353581#:~:text=A%20core%20body%20temperature%
     20of,can%20all%20result%20from%20heatstroke.

139 the threshold at which heat-related illness begins: Roxana Chicas

et al., "Cooling Interventions Among Agricultural Workers: A Pilot Study," *Workplace Health and Safety* 69, no. 7 (2020): 315–22, doi .org/10.1177/2165079920976524.

139 Roxana Chicas, PhD, RN: All quotes from and information about Roxana Chicas, including the description of her work in Florida, are from both phone and in-person interviews, August 13, 2020; July 13–14, 2021; and May 6, 2022.

139 for every five-degree increase in the heat index: Jacqueline Mix et al., "Hydration Status, Kidney Function, and Kidney Injury in Florida Agricultural Workers," *Journal of Occupational and Environmental Medicine* 60, no. 5 (2018): e253, doi.org/10.1097/jom.0000000000001261.

140 regular access to water, rest, and shade: "New Study Shows Heat Stress Protections Prevent Kidney Injury Among Farmworkers—and Save Lives," *Farmworker Justice* (blog), n.d., www.farmworkerjustice.org/blog-post /new-study-shows-heat-stress-protections-prevent-kidney-injury -among-farmworkers-and-save-lives/.

142 twenty times more likely to die of heat stroke: "Heat-Related Deaths Among Crop Workers—United States, 1992–2006," Centers for Disease Control and Prevention, n.d., www.cdc.gov/mmwr/preview/mmwrht ml/mm5724a1.htm.

142 thirteen times more likely to die from heat stroke: Payel Acharya, Bethany Boggess, and Kai Zhang, "Assessing Heat Stress and Health Among Construction Workers in a Changing Climate: A Review," *International Journal of Environmental Research and Public Health* 15, no. 2 (2018): 247, doi.org/10.3390/ijerph15020247.

142 Washington State has temporary emergency laws in effect: Bridget Huber, "As Heat Rises, Who Will Protect Farmworkers?" *Mother Jones*, July 1, 2022, www.motherjones.com/food/2022/07/as-heat-rises-who -will-protect-farmworkers/.

142 temperature that day was over one hundred degrees: Katherine Cook, "Oregon Farm Worker Dies During Heat Wave," KGW, June 29, 2021, www.kgw.com/article/news/local/oregon-farm-worker-dies-heat-wave -pacific-northwest/283–85b9cb18–4c17–435a–8a7c–3efce4f6545d; Monica Samayoa, "Oregon OSHA Enacts Temporary Rules, but Some Worry If They Go Far Enough," OPB, July 9, 2021, www.opb.org/article /2021/07/08/oregon-osha-enacts-temporary-rules-workers/.

143 It does: Roxana Chicas et al., "Hydration Interventions Among Agricul-

tural Workers: A Pilot Study," *Journal of Occupational and Environmental Medicine* 64, no. 5 (2022):doi.org/10.1097/jom.0000000000002531.

143 accurately measure: Yun Soung Kim et al., "Soft Wireless Bioelectronics Designed for Real Time, Continuous Health Monitoring of Farmworkers," *Advanced Healthcare Materials* 11, no. 13 (2022): 2200170, doi.org/10.1002/adhm.202200170.

144 gesturing to the busy room: I was observing with two Spanish interpreters, who translated for me, with the consent of participants.

145 running the infirmary at her monastery: Victoria Sweet, "Hildegard of Bingen and the Greening of Medieval Medicine," *Bulletin of the History of Medicine* 73, no. 3 (1999): 397, doi.org/10.1353/bhm.1999.0140.

146 "that stuffiness in his head will diminish": Hildegard von Bingen, trans. Priscilla Throop, *Hildegard von Bingen's "Physica": The Complete English Translation of Her Classic Work on Health and Healing* (Rochester, VT: Healing Arts Press, 1998), 22.

146 "causes them to be moved and to emit sparks": von Bingen, *Causes and Cures*, 12.

146 only when the environmental elements were in balance: Sweet, "Hildegard of Bingen and the Greening of Medieval Medicine," 388–89.

147 "'There's something more we can do'": Potter author interview.

147 Haas-Howard, MPH, RN: Christy Haas-Howard, Zoom author interview, June 14, 2021.

147 at some public schools, 20 to 30 percent of all kids: Kati Weis, "Many Denver Schools with High Asthma Rates Aren't Participating in a New Air Quality Monitoring Program," Chalkbeat Colorado, July 12, 2019, co.chalkbeat.org/2019/7/12/21108548/many-denver-schools-with-high-asthma-rates-aren-t-participating-in-a-new-air-quality-monitoring-prog.

147 bad air quality, which comes with climate change: "Asthma in the US," Centers for Disease Control and Prevention, updated May 3, 2011, www.cdc.gov/vitalsigns/asthma/index.html#:~:text=Asthma%20is%20increasing%20every%20year%20in%20the%20US.&text=More%20children%20(57%25)%20than,than%20girls%20to%20have%20asthma.

148 Jessica LeClair, MPH, RN: Jessica LeClair, telephone interview with author, August 4, 2020.

150 Katie Huffling, DNP, RN: Huffling author interview, June 8, 2021.

CHAPTER 8: ADDICTION

153 Jason Fox, NP: All quotes from and information about Jason Fox are from Zoom author interview, March 17, 2022.

154 A 2012 study found: Deborah S. Finnell, "A Clarion Call for Nurse-Led SBIRT Across the Continuum of Care," *Alcoholism: Clinical and Experimental Research* 36, no. 7 (2012): 1134–38, https://doi.org/10.1111/j.15 30–0277.2012.01870.x.

155 alcohol- and drug overdose–related deaths: "Alcohol Deaths on the Rise and Suicide Declines," Centers for Disease Control and Prevention, March 18, 2022, www.cdc.gov/nchs/pressroom/podcasts/2022 /20220318/20220318.htm.

155 continue to rise: National Institute on Drug Abuse, "Overdose Death Rates," U.S. Department of Health and Human Services, January 20, 2022, nida.nih.gov/research-topics/trends-statistics/overdose-death-rates.

155 are higher now than ever before: Deidre McPhillips, "In 2021, US Drug Overdose Deaths Hit Highest Level on Record, CDC Data Shows," CNN, May 11, 2022, www.cnn.com/2022/05/11/health/drug -overdose-deaths-record-high-2021/index.html.

158 the virus that caused AIDS was spreading: "Evolution of Harm Reduction," National Harm Reduction Coalition, May 12, 2022, harmreduc tion.org/movement/evolution/.

158 development of maintenance medications like methadone: Christine Vestal, "Long Stigmatized, Methadone Clinics Multiply in Some States," Pew Charitable Trusts, www.pewtrusts.org/en/research-and-analysis /blogs/stateline/2018/10/31/long-stigmatized-methadone-clinics-multi ply-in-some-states.

159 called *Afyunieh*: Abdolali Moosavyzadeh et al., "The Medieval Persian Manuscript of *Afyunieh*: The First Individual Treatise on the Opium and Addiction in History," *Journal of Integrative Medicine* 16, no. 2 (2018): 77–83, doi.org/10.1016/j.joim.2018.02.004.

159 L. Synn Stern, MPH, RN: All quotes and information about L. Synn Stern are from in-person author interview, March 31, 2022.

160 One afternoon in March: All descriptions of the safe consumption room are from in-person author visit to New York Harm Reduction Educators offices, March 31, 2022.

160 detox program developed by the Young Lords: *Dope Is Death*, directed

by Mia Donovan (EyeSteelFilm, 2020), www.eyesteelfilm.com/port folio/dopeisdeath.

163 like Philadelphia: Nina Feldman, "In Philadelphia, Judges Rule Against Opening 'Supervised' Site to Inject Opioids," NPR, January 14, 2021, www.npr.org/sections/health-shots/2021/01/14/956428659/in-phila delphia-judges-rule-against-opening-a-medical-site-to-safely-inject -hero.

164 syringe exchange in Harlem and the Bronx: "About-History," New York Harm Reduction Educators, October 11, 2016, nyhre.org/about/.

164 he also handed out mittens, cookies, and condoms: Jane Gross, "Needle Exchange for Addicts Wins Foothold Against AIDS in Tacoma," New York Times, January 23, 1989, www.nytimes.com/1989/01/23/us /needle-exchange-for-addicts-wins-foothold-against-aids-in-tacoma .html.

164 Syringe exchange programs worked: Mireya Navarro, "New York Needle Exchanges Called Surprisingly Effective," New York Times, February 18, 1993, www.nytimes.com/1993/02/18/nyregion/new-york-need le-exchanges-called-surprisingly-effective.html.

164 legalized in New York State, which was around 1992: National Research Council and Institute of Medicine Panel on Needle Exchange and Bleach Distribution Programs, Proceedings Workshop on Needle Exchange and Bleach Distribution Programs (Washington, DC: National Academies Press, 1994, www.ncbi.nlm.nih.gov/books/NBK23 6642/.

164 fell from 50 percent to 17 percent: "Access to Clean Syringes," Centers for Disease Control and Prevention, August 5, 2016, www.cdc.gov /policy/hst/hi5/cleansyringes/index.html.

167 official policy: Martha Bebinger, "Drug Overdose Deaths Are at a Record High. Here's What the White House Plans to Do," NPR, April 21, 2022, www.npr.org/2022/04/21/1093974276/drug-overdose-deaths-opi oid-fentanyl.

167 accidental overdoses that are so common now: Andrew Joseph, "'This Program's Really Saved Us': As Canada Offers Safer Opioids to Curb Overdoses, Will U.S. Follow?" STAT, September 21, 2022, www.statnews .com/2022/09/21/canada-giving-out-safer-opioids-to-stem-overdoses -will-u-s-follow/.

167 7.1 percent of both Black and Hispanic people: Substance Abuse and Mental Health Services Administration "Racial/Ethnic Differences in Substance Use, Substance Use Disorders, and Substance Use Treatment Utilization Among People Aged 12 or Older," SAMHSA, 2021, www.samhsa.gov/data/report/racialethnic-differences-substance-use.

168 overdose deaths of white Americans have sharply risen: "Opioid Overdose Deaths by Race/Ethnicity," Table, Kaiser Family Foundation, May 9, 2022, www.kff.org/other/state-indicator/opioid-overdose-deaths-by-raceethnicity/.

CHAPTER 9: COLLECTIVE

169 Lavinia L. Dock, RN: Lavinia L. Dock, "Status of the Nurse in the Working World," *American Journal of Nursing* 13, no. 12 (1913): 971, https://doi.org/10.1097/00000446-191309000-00021.

169 went to war against Governor Arnold Schwarzenegger: Zoom author interview with Gerard Brogan, August 3, 2022.

170 "I'm always kicking their butt": "Schwarzenegger Provokes Nurses' Wrath," *Nursing Standard* 19, no. 22 (2005): 5, doi.org/10.7748/ns.19.22.5.s9.

170 "If you're a patient's advocate": Ina Jaffe, "The Political Clout of California's Nurses," NPR, August 8, 2006, www.npr.org/templates/story/story.php?storyId=5627701.

170 flew a blimp over his house: Mark Martin, "Nurses Take Special Interest in Governor; Battle Heats Up Between Union, Schwarzenegger," *San Francisco Chronicle*, February 26, 2005, www.sfgate.com/health/article/Nurses-take-special-interest-in-governor-Battle-2695818.php.

171 Gerard Brogan, RN,: Zoom interview with the author, August 3, 2022.

171 a branch of the American Nurses Association: "About CNA," National Nurses United, December 23, 2021, www.nationalnursesunited.org/about-cna.

172 things were very bad: Cara S. Lesser, Paul B. Ginsburg, and Kelly J. Devers, "The End of an Era: What Became of the 'Managed Care Revolution' in 2001?" *Health Services Research* 38, no. 1, pt. 2 (2003): 337–55, www.ncbi.nlm.nih.gov/pmc/articles/PMC1360889/.

173 discharged alive: Linda H. Aiken et al., "Hospital Nurse Staffing and Patient Mortality, Nurse Burnout, and Job Dissatisfaction." *JAMA* 288, no. 16 (2002): 1987–93, doi:10.1001/jama.288.16.1987.

Linda H. Aiken et al., "Implications of the California Nurse Staffing Mandate for Other States," *Health Services Research* 45, no. 4 (2010): 904–21, www.ncbi.nlm.nih.gov/pmc/articles/PMC2908200/.

173 in court: Carolyn Marshall, "Schwarzenegger Abandons Court Fight Against Nurses," *New York Times*, November 12, 2005, www.nytimes .com/2005/11/12/us/schwarzenegger-abandons-court-fight-against -nurses.html.

173 into the 30s: Ed Leibowitz, "The Man Who Tried to Make California Great Again," *Los Angeles Magazine*, November 11, 2016, www.lamag .com/longform/the-rise-and-fall-of-governor-arnold-schwarze/.

173 playing "nice": Debra Jackson, "When Niceness Becomes Toxic, or How Niceness Effectively Silences Nurses and Maintains the Status Quo in Nursing," *Journal of Advanced Nursing* 78, no. 10 (2022): doi.org/10 .1111/jan.15407.

174 duties, not rights: Reverby, *Ordered to Care*, 2.

174 close to zero: Reverby, *Ordered to Care*, 61.

174 essentially for free: Jean C. Whelan, "Surpluses, Shortages, and Segrega- tion," in her *Nursing the Nation, Building the Nurse Labor Force* (New Brunswick, NJ: Rutgers University Press, 2021), chap. 4, 67–87.

174 nursing workforce: Whelan, "Surpluses, Shortages, and Segregation," 67–87.

174 nurses who would work for free: Whelan, "Surpluses, Shortages, and Segregation," 67–87.

175 became more and more the norm: Whelan, "More and More (and Bet- ter) Nurses," 142.

176 hospital groups: "Facts Matter on Staffing Ratios," CEO Message, Cal- ifornia Hospital Association, March 11, 2021, calhospital.org/facts -matter-staffing-ratios/.

176 to meet the ratio law's staffing requirements: Marshall, "Schwarzeneg- ger Abandons Court Fight Against Nurses."

176 increased when the law went into effect: Roxanne Nelson, "California's Ratio Law, Four Years Later," *AJN, American Journal of Nursing* 108, no. 3 (2008): 25–26, doi.org/10.1097/01.naj.0000312244.28680.93.

176 a concurrent rise in salaries: Aiken, et al., "Implications of the California Nurse Staffing Mandate for Other States."

176 or health care workers generally: M. Nielsen, D. D'Agostino, and P. Greg- ory, "Addressing Rural Health Challenges Head On," *Missouri Medicine*

114, no. 5 (Sept.–Oct. 2017): 363–66, www.ncbi.nlm.nih.gov/pmc/arti cles/PMC6140198/.

176 to go around: Aallyah Wright, "Rural Hospitals Can't Find the Nurses They Need to Fight COVID," Pew Charitable Trusts, September 1, 2021, www.pewtrusts.org/en/research-and-analysis/blogs/stateline/2021 /09/01/rural-hospitals-cant-find-the-nurses-they-need-to-fight-covid.

176 Patrick McMurray, MSN, RN: Patrick McMurray, "We Have Shortage of Nurses Who Come from Historically Excluded Groups in Nursing as a Whole and Even More Severely in the Areas of Nursing Research /Academia, Faculty, and Leadership," tweet, Twitter, July 28, 2022, twitter.com/NursePatMacRN/status/1552757217849401344.

176 retiring just as demand for nurses is increasing: "The Aging Nursing Workforce," Simmons University, May 13, 2021, online.simmons.edu /blog/aging-nursing-workforce/.

176 no large nationwide shortage of nurses this decade: J. L. Flaubert et al., eds., National Academies of Sciences, Engineering, and Medicine; National Academy of Medicine; Committee on the Future of Nursing 2020–2030, "The Nursing Workforce," part 3 of *The Future of Nursing 2020–2030: Charting a Path to Achieve Health Equity* (Washington, DC: National Academies Press, 2021), www.ncbi.nlm.nih.gov/books /NBK573922/.

176 4.4 million currently licensed registered nurses: National Council of State Boards of Nursing, "Active RN Licenses."

177 60 percent of those in inpatient hospitals: U.S. Bureau of Labor Statistics, "Registered Nurses."

177 by rates of 30 to 57 percent: "Recruiting and Retaining New Nurse Grads," Wolters Kluwer, October 19, 2017, www.wolterskluwer.com/en /expert-insights/recruiting-retaining-new-nurse-grads.

178 actively opposed by the American Nurses Association: Massachusetts Hospital Association. ANA Massachusetts Announces Opposition to Nurse Staffing Ballot Question. Accessed November 18, 2022. https:// www.mhalink.org/MHA/MyMHA/Communications/PressReleases /Content/2018/ANA_MassAnnouncesOpposition_toNurseStaffing BallotQuestion.aspx.

179 put on furlough or laid off: Soumya Karlamangla and Melanie Mason, "Thousands of Healthcare Workers Are Laid Off or Furloughed as Coronavirus Spreads," *Los Angeles Times*, May 3, 2020, www.latimes.com

/california/story/2020–05–02/coronavirus-california-healthcare-work
ers-layoffs-furloughs.

179 by some accounts: Shannon Firth, "Nurses Report Continued Mental Health Issues for Third Year in a Row," Medical News, MedpageToday, July 26, 2022, www.medpagetoday.com/hospitalbasedmedicine/nurs ing/99898.

179 Cortney, a registered nurse: Cortney, author phone interview, April 21, 2020.

180 Tiffany: Tiffany, author phone interview, July 29, 2022.

182 the Christian disease: M. Tampa, "Brief History of Syphilis," *Journal of Medicine and Life* 7, no. 1 (March 2014): 4–10, www.ncbi.nlm.nih.gov /pmc/articles/PMC3956094/.

182 Francesca: Sharon T. Strocchia, "Restoring Health," in her *Forgotten Healers*, chap. 5, 191.

182 "moral agents who offset the effects of sexual vice": Strocchia, "Restoring Health," 191.

183 congressional investigation into travel nursing's high wages: Sarah Di-Gregorio, "Hospitals Desperately Need Staff, but Capping Travel Nurses' Pay Won't Help," *Washington Post*, March 14, 2022, www.washing tonpost.com/outlook/2022/03/14/travel-nurse-pay-caps/.

184 about five thousand: "About the AHA," American Hospital Association, n.d., www.aha.org/about.

184 "Hospitals also have incurred significant costs in recruiting": "Data Brief: Workforce Issues Remain at the Forefront of Pandemic," American Hospital Association, January 2022, www.aha.org/system/files /media/file/2022/01/Data-Brief-Workforce-Issues-012422.pdf/.

184 stressful work environments and inadequate staffing: Megha K. Shah, "Prevalence of and Factors Associated with Nurse Burnout in the US," *JAMA Network Open* 4, no. 2 (2021), doi.org/10.1001/jamanetwork open.2020.36469.

184 over thirty million dollars in 2020: Hannah Mitchell, "The 7 Highest-Paid Health System CEOS," Becker's Hospital Review, n.d., beckers hospitalreview.com/rankings-and-ratings/the-7-highest-paid-health -system-ceos.html?oly_enc_id=7598I1302867J9X.

184 value to the community: Karen E. Joynt, "Compensation of Chief Executive Officers at Nonprofit US Hospitals," *JAMA Internal Medicine* 174, no. 1 (2014): 61, doi.org/10.1001/jamainternmed.2013.11537.

185 won it: Aparna Gopalan, "Massachusetts Nurses Just Won an Epic 10-Month Strike," The New Republic, November 18, 2022, https://new republic.com/article/164950/st-vincent-hospital-nurses-strike.

185 a dispute that is ongoing: "Why 15,000 Nurses Went on Strike in Minnesota," PBS, September 18, 2022, www.pbs.org/newshour/show/why -15000-nurses-went-on-strike-in-minnesota.

185 Erin, an ICU nurse: Erin, author Zoom interview, January 10, 2022.

CHAPTER 10: POWER

187 Phara Souffrant Forrest, BSN, RN: All information and quotes from Phara Souffrant Forrest are from author phone interview, February 2, 2022.

189 a thirty-five-dollar monthly cap on insulin costs: "Cori Bush and Democrats Finalizing a Plan to Lower Insulin Costs," More Perfect Union, November 12, 2021, perfectunion.us/cori-bush-insulin-costs/.

189 to all: Rachel Pannett and Rachel Roubein. "The GOP Blocked an Insulin Price Cap: What It Means for Diabetics," The Washington Post, WP Company, August 9, 2022, https://www.washingtonpost.com/health /2022/08/08/insulin-price-cap-diabetes-senate-republicans/.

189 the fact that health care is a human right: "Congresswoman Bush Leads First Oversight Hearing on Medicare for All," Cori Bush Congresswoman for Missouri's 1st, March 30, 2022, bush.house.gov/media /press-releases/congresswoman-bush-leads-first-oversight-hearing-on -medicare-for-all.

189 winning by 60 percentage points in 2020: Bruce Handy, "Cori Bush, a Nurse and Activist, Becomes the First Black Woman to Represent Missouri in Congress," The New Yorker, November 7, 2020, www.newyork er.com/magazine/2020/11/16/cori-bush-becomes-first-black-woman -and-first-nurse-to-represent-missouri-in-congress.

189 two newly elected Wisconsin assemblypersons: Anthony Dabruzzi, "Two Nurses Become State Lawmakers amid a Pandemic," Spectrum News 1, May 7 2021, spectrumnews1.com/wi/madison/politics/2021/05/07/two -nurses-become-state-lawmakers-amid-a-pandemic.

189 yearly Gallup poll: Kathleen Gaines, "Nursing Ranked as the Most Trusted Profession for 20th Year in a Row," Nurse.org, n.d., nurse.org /articles/nursing-ranked-most-honest-profession/.

190 wrote a letter to the editor: Lavinia Dock, "The Suffrage Question," Amer-

ican Journal of Nursing 8, no. 11 (August 1908): 925–26, http://doi
.org/10.1097/00000446-190808000-00021.

191 too divisive: Ernest J. Grant, PhD, RN, FAAN, "An Open Letter to the
ANA Membership," Capitol Beat, American Nurses Association, September 15, 2020, anacapitolbeat.org/2020/09/15/an-open-letter-to-the
-ana-membership/.

191 Lavinia Dock was born into: Biographical details throughout are from
Mary E. Garofalo and Elizabeth Fee, "Lavinia Dock (1858–1956): Picketing, Parading, and Protesting," *American Journal of Public Health* 105,
no. 2 (2015): 276–77, doi.org/10.2105/ajph.2014.302021; and "Lavinia
Lloyd Dock," American Association for the History of Nursing, n.d.,
www.aahn.org/dock.

192 dedicated herself to women's suffrage: For Dock's political activities,
see Carole A. Estabrooks, "Lavinia Lloyd Dock: The Henry Street Years,"
Nursing History Review 3, no. 1 (1995): 143–72, connect.springerpub
.com/content/sgrnhr/3/1/143; Phoebe Pollitt, "Nurses Fight for the
Right to Vote," *American Journal of Nursing* 118, no. 11 (2018): 46–49,
doi.org/10.1097/01.naj.0000547639.70037.cd; and Mary Lou Schwartz,
"Lavinia Dock: Adams County Suffragette–Gettysburg College," Adams County History, 1997, cupola.gettysburg.edu/cgi/viewcontent.cgi
?httpsredir=1&article=1016&context=ach.

192 "to retain the possession of her banner": United Press, "Miss Lavinia
Dock Seized with Pickets: Former Harrisburg Woman Fights Policeman
to Retain Banner: Lively Struggle Near White House," *Evening News*,
June 26, 1917.

192 force-fed raw eggs: Catharine Hamm, "In 1917, the 'Night of Terror' at
a Virginia Prison Changed History. Now It's a Site of Beauty," *Los Angeles Times*, November 12, 2017, www.latimes.com/travel/la-tr-woman
-occoquan-20171112-htmlstory.html.

192 "It was a great joy to do a little guerilla war": Lavinia L. Dock, "Lavinia
L. Dock: Self Portrait," *Nursing Outlook* 25, no. 1 (January 1977): 56,
pubmed.ncbi.nlm.nih.gov/319427/.

192 she wrote: Dock "Status of the Nurse in the Working World," 975.

193 when she was just fourteen: Raina Lipsitz, "The Resilience of India
Walton," *The Nation*, September 15, 2021, www.thenation.com/article
/politics/buffalo-mayor-india-walton/.

193 truest role of a nurse is advocate: Unless otherwise noted, all quotes by

and information about India Walton are from in-person author interview, November 22, 2021.

196 former governor Andrew Cuomo: Zack Fink, "Hochul Stands by Jacobs, Won't Endorse Democratic Nominee in Buffalo Mayor's Race," Spectrum News 1, October 23, 2022, www.ny1.com/nyc/all-boroughs/news/2021/10/19/hochul-stands-by-jacobs—won-t-endorse-democratic-nominee-in-buffalo-mayor-s-race.

196 Tarik S. Khan, PhD, CRNP: Tarik Khan, author Zoom interview, May 26, 2022.

196 prevailed in an underdog win: Lizzy McLellan Ravitch, and Asha Prihar, "Philly's State Legislative Races Were Kind of Wild This Year, but the Primary Ended up Bringing Few Surprises," Billy Penn, May 18, 2022, billypenn.com/2022/05/17/midterm-primary-results-philadelphia-pennsylvania-house-senate-democrats/.

196 driving around Philadelphia giving out vaccines: Marilyn D. Harris, "A Day in the Life of a COVID Vaccine Champion," *Home Healthcare Now* 39, no. 6 (2021): 357, doi.org/10.1097/nhh.0000000000001016.

199 minimum wage: "New York State's Minimum Wage," The State of New York, n.d., www.ny.gov/new-york-states-minimum-wage/new-york-states-minimum-wage.

199 in 2022: "The New York State Department of Labor Announces Minimum Wage Increase for Home Care Aides," Department of Labor. Accessed November 18, 2022. dol.ny.gov/news/new-york-state-department-labor-announces-minimum-wage-increase-home-care-aides#:~:text=Effective%20October%201%2C%202022%2C%20through,remainder%20of%20New%20York%20State.

EPILOGUE: LOVE IN ACTION

202 LeBeau graduated from nursing school: All information on and quotes by Marcella LeBeau are from in-person author interview, June 2, 2021.

202 Cheyenne River Sioux Tribe: "History: Cheyenne River Sioux Tribe: Eagle Butte," CRST, n.d., www.cheyenneriversiouxtribe.org/history.

206 "Kill the Indian, save the man": Staff, Native News Online, "NCAI Weighs in on Discovery of Remains of 215 Children at Indian Residential School in Canada," Native News Online, June 3, 2021, nativenews online.net/currents/ncai-weighs-in-on-discovery-of-remains-of-215-children-at-indian-residential-school-in-canada.

206 hundreds of thousands of Native or Indigenous children: "US Indian Boarding School History," The National Native American Boarding School Healing Coalition, n.d., boardingschoolhealing.org/education/us-indian-boarding-school-history/.

209 Young people, parents with small children, die at a devastating rate: Kayla Gahagan, "On Reservation, Hope Remains Despite Grim Statistics," WebMD, November 1, 2018, www.webmd.com/healthy-aging/news/20181101/on-reservation-hope-remains-despite-grim-statistics; "About the Pine Ridge Reservation," Re-Member, n.d., www.re-member.org/pine-ridge-reservation.

210 "by all people": "Why 'Caring Matters Most.'" Yale School of Nursing, February 14, 2017, https://nursing.yale.edu/news/why-caring-matters-most.

SELECTED BIBLIOGRAPHY

Baptiste, Diana Lyn, et al. "Hidden Figures of Nursing: The Historical Contributions of Black Nurses and a Narrative for Those Who Are Unnamed, Undocumented, and Underrepresented." *Journal of Advanced Nursing* 77, no. 4 (2021): 1627-32. doi.org/10.1111/jan.14791.

D'Antonio, Patricia. *American Nursing: A History of Knowledge, Authority, and the Meaning of Work.* Baltimore, MD: Johns Hopkins University Press, 2010.

Eisler, Riane, et al. *Transforming Interprofessional Partnerships: A New Framework for Nursing and Partnership-Based Health Care.* Indianapolis, IN: Sigma Theta Tau International, 2014.

Fett, Sharla M. *Working Cures: Healing, Health, and Power on Southern Slave Plantations.* Chapel Hill: University of North Carolina Press, 2002.

Helmstadter, Carol. *Beyond Nightingale: Nursing on the Crimean War Battlefields.* Manchester, UK: Manchester University Press, 2021.

Hine, Darlene Clark. *Black Women in White Racial Conflict and Cooperation in the Nursing Profession, 1890-1950.* Bloomington, IN: Indiana University Press, 1989.

Lazenby, Mark. *Caring Matters Most: The Ethical Significance of Nursing.* New York: Oxford University Press, 2017.

Lazenby, Mark. *Toward a Better World: The Social Significance of Nursing.* New York: Oxford University Press, 2020.

Mitchem, Stephanie Y. *African American Folk Healing.* New York: New York University Press, 2007.

Nutting, M. Adelaide, and Lavinia L. Dock. *A History of Nursing.* Vol. 1. New York: G.P. Putnam's Sons, 1907.

Reverby, Susan. *Ordered to Care: The Dilemma of American Nursing, 1850–1945*. Cambridge, UK: Cambridge University Press, 2004.

Risse, Guenter B. *Mending Bodies, Saving Souls: A History of Hospitals*. New York: Oxford University Press, 1999.

Ritchey, Sara Margaret. *Acts of Care: Recovering Women in Late Medieval Health*. Ithaca, NY: Cornell University Press, 2021.

Seacole, Mary, and Sara Salih. *Wonderful Adventures of Mrs Seacole in Many Lands*. London: Penguin, 2005.

Smith, Kylie M., et al. "Moving Beyond Florence: Why We Need to Decolonize Nursing History." Nursing Clio, February 4, 2021. nursingclio.org/topics/beyond-florence/.

Staupers, M. Keaton. *No Time for Prejudice*. New York: Macmillan, 1961.

Strocchia, Sharon T. *Forgotten Healers: Women and the Pursuit of Health in Late Renaissance Italy*. Cambridge, Massachusetts; London: Harvard University Press, 2019.

Threat, Charissa J. *Nursing Civil Rights: Gender and Race in the Army Nurse Corps*. Urbana: University of Illinois Press, 2015.

Valdez, Anna. "Leading Change in the International Year of the Nurse and Midwife." *Teaching and Learning in Nursing* 15, no. 2 (2020): A2-A4. doi.org/10.1016/j.teln.2020.01.003.

Wald, Lillian D. *The House on Henry Street . . . with Illustrations, Etc.* New York: Henry Holt and Company, 1915.

Whelan, Jean C. *Nursing the Nation: Building the Nurse Labor Force*. New Brunswick, NJ: Rutgers University Press, 2021.

INDEX

ABOUT THE AUTHOR

SARAH DiGREGORIO is the author of *Early: An Intimate History of Premature Birth and What It Teaches Us About Being Human*. She is a freelance journalist who has written on health care and other topics for the *New York Times*, the *Washington Post*, the *Wall Street Journal*, *Slate*, *Insider*, and *Catapult*. She lives in Brooklyn, New York, with her daughter and husband.

Read More by Sarah DiGregorio

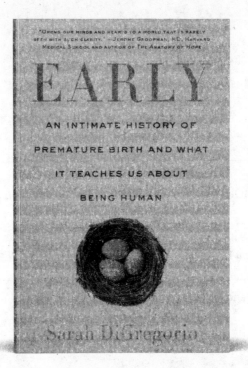

"The heart of DiGregorio's illuminating book isn't just about her family's journey; it's an expansive examination of the history and ethics of neonatology." —*New York Times Book Review*

"A sweeping cultural history, a consistently surprising and insightful examination on the porous line between life and death, and a graceful and hauntingly clear-eyed memoir all in one. Feels destined to live on shelves for a long time."
—**Jayson Greene, author of *Once More We Saw Stars***

HARPER

HarperCollins*Publishers*

Discover great authors, exclusive offers, and more at HC.com.